WORKING WITH GROUPS TO EXPLORE

Food & *Body*

CONNECTIONS

WORKING WITH GROUPS TO EXPLORE

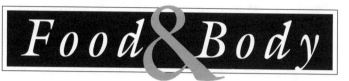

Food & Body

CONNECTIONS

Eating Issues ■ *Body Image*
Size Acceptance ■ *Self-Care*

Sandy Stewart Christian, MSW   Editor

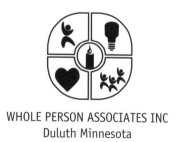

WHOLE PERSON ASSOCIATES INC
Duluth Minnesota

REPRODUCTION POLICY

Unless otherwise noted, your purchase of this volume entitles you to reproduce a modest quantity of the worksheets that appear in this book for your education/ training activities. For this limited worksheet reproduction, no special additional permission is needed. However the following statement, in total, must appear on all copies that you reproduce.

> Reproduced from *Working with Groups to Explore Food & Body Connections,* Sandy Stewart Christian, ed. © 1996 Whole Person Associates Inc, 210 West Michigan, Duluth MN 55802.

Specific prior written permission is required from the publisher for any reproduction of a complete or adapted exercise with trainer instructions, or large-scale reproduction of worksheets, or for inclusion of material in another publication. Licensing or royalty arrangement requests for this usage must be submitted in writing and approved prior to any such use.

For further information, please write for our Permissions Guidelines and Standard Permissions Form. Permission requests must be submitted at least thirty days in advance of your scheduled printing or reproduction.

Library of Congress Cataloging in Publication Data
Working with groups to explore food & body connections / Sandy Stewart Christian, editor.
      208p. 23cm. — (Structured exercises in healing)
      Includes bibliographical references.
      ISBN 1-57025-105-3
      1. Eating disorders—Prevention. 2. Group counseling. 3. Nutrition—Psychological aspects. 4. Body image. 5. Food habits. I. Christian, Sandy Stewart. II. Series.
RC552.E18W67   1996
616.85' 2605—dc20   95-49465
                                                                      CIP

Printed in the United States of America

10 9 8 7 6 5 4 3 2 1

WHOLE PERSON ASSOCIATES INC
210 West Michigan
Duluth MN 55802
(800) 247-6789

PREFACE

One of the joyful things about working on this project has been the contacts with contributors, who have been most generous in sharing creative ideas, time, energy, and other resources that have enriched and broadened the scope of the book. It was heartwarming to make new connections with professionals of varied backgrounds from around the country, all of whom are working in the field to promote healthy food and body connections.

As a systems-thinker with a whole person focus, I am always appreciative of the power of a group to create something that goes beyond the original concept or plan, and turn it into a process that takes on a life of its own. This book was the outgrowth of several group support systems.

I am grateful to the diverse group of professional women in Duluth who participated in focus groups, shaped the concept of this book, and built a solid foundation for its overall content. These consultants included a registered nurse, a nurse practitioner, dietitians, weight management program staff and directors, an occupational therapist, college educators, clinical social workers, health educators, and licensed psychologists. All of these women work with eating disorders or other food/body problems in a wide variety of settings: hospitals, eating disorder treatment programs, inpatient and outpatient mental health programs, medical clinics, private therapy practice groups, and colleges and universities. I want to thank Roxanne Bijold, Mary Graff, Chris Henley, Nancy Hinzman, Gayle Potter, Yvonne Prettner, Mary Martin, Pam Solberg-Tapper, Katherine Speare, and Ruth Strom McCutcheon for their participation in the focus group and for the wealth of experience and ideas they contributed to this project. Nancy Tubesing was a dynamic facilitator of the focus group, and Heather Isernhagen was a diligent recorder.

My personal support group of the past fifteen years has made invaluable contributions toward my personal growth and the process of making peace with food and my own body. The collective wisdoms of Nancy, Mary G., Mary M., Gloria, and Ruth are an integral part of me, and this book.

The Whole Person Associates and Pfeifer-Hamilton Publishers staff have always provided a supportive, nurturing environment in which to work. I appreciate the efforts of each person who helped move this book to completion. A special thanks goes to Heather for her work at the computer, to Sally for her wonderful artistic design, and to Nancy for her creative visioning, editing, mentoring, and ongoing support.

I want to thank my own family, Don, Paul, and Jenna, for their loving support throughout this project. They are the ultimate support group.

Duluth MN   Sandy Stewart Christian
October 1995

v

TABLE OF CONTENTS

INTRODUCTION

All of us are concerned to a greater or lesser degree by what we eat, how we look, and how we feel about ourselves. A few people never struggle with eating or body image issues. Some become totally obsessed by food or the search for a perfect body. The rest of us fall somewhere in between.

Ideally, we would all naturally enjoy peaceful, pleasurable, healthy styles of eating, and each of us would care lovingly for her body. Unfortunately, for many people, attaining or maintaining a healthy body weight is a constant struggle. Food is something to fear, eating is a source of confusion and conflict, and body image is a focus of painful self-deprecation. Why is this so, and what can we do to help?

If you are a wellness educator, health professional, program developer, consultant, behaviorist, trainer, growth/support group leader, therapist, nutritionist, dietitian, fitness or recreational director, occupational therapist, or other group leader interested in helping people explore their food and body connections, this book is for you.

This book is a collection of 36 structured exercises on a wide range of food and body-related topics, written for diverse audiences, in a variety of settings. There are processes suited for workplace wellness programs, community education, weight management programs, ongoing growth and support groups, treatment groups, therapy groups, and professional education groups. The presentations and activities were developed for people who need to lose weight for health reasons, women (and men) who want to stop dieting but don't know what to do instead, overeaters who want a normal relationship with food, individuals in recovery from eating disorders, and anyone else seeking a healthier food and body connection.

WHO MIGHT USE THIS BOOK?

Wellness educators will find group processes that stimulate reflection and problem solving about unhealthy styles of eating and exercising. *Consultants* and *trainers* will find ideas for exploring eating habits, body image, values, and cultural bias. *Nutritionists* and *weight-management counselors* will find practical ideas for helping people explore relationships with food and choose satisfying, healthful food at the supermarket. *Support group leaders* will find playful ways to challenge fat-ism and promote size acceptance. And *therapists* will be able to use many processes to help people heal from negative body image, break free from compulsive eating, and recover from life-threatening eating disorders.

The exercises in this book reflect a diverse, multidimensional view of food and body problems, and a holistic approach to understanding and helping people who are struggling with eating, weight, and body issues. The whole person perspective assumes that the whole person—mind, body, and spirit, in context with the social and cultural environment—is dynamically involved with any health issue, including food and body balance. When we work with groups on such intimate issues as food and body concerns, it is helpful to explore the way all these dimensions affect a person's life or total well-being.

The contributors to this book represent this diversity and bring a wide variety of experiences and perspectives to this book. Many are leaders in the new wave of health education that focuses on health and fitness for *all* sizes, instead of only the thin. They include pioneers in the wellness movement, writers and researchers, consultants, nutritionists, dietitians, physicians, dancers, aerobics instructors, artists, workshop leaders, spiritual directors, clergy, health educators, social workers, psychologists, psychoanalysts, behaviorists in weight-management programs, college faculty, marriage and family therapists, program developers, and support group leaders.

WHAT ARE THE ISSUES?

While food and body conflicts affect all people in our culture, there are special issues for women who suffer in alarming rates from negative body image (even body hatred), food and weight obsessions, eating disorders, and chronic dieting. Something is wrong when the majority of 10-year-old girls in the United States are already on diets or think they are the ugliest girl in their 4th grade class. Something is wrong when 75% of American women think they are too fat, when 25% of college women are bulimic, and when less than 50% of women will say, "I like my body the way it is." Something is wrong when, on any given day, 48 million girls and women are on a diet and when 33 billion dollars are spent annually on diets or diet products, in spite of the research that clearly demonstrates the failure of traditional diets as a means of achieving a healthy, stable weight.

Cultural standards of beauty and worth are, for women, superficial. The measuring stick is often appearance—how we look in shorts, how we compare with the models in magazines—not how we function in the world or the contributions we make to society. For many women, this social conditioning is at the root of their conflicts with food and their body.

Men also have issues related to food and body image. Athletes, body builders, fitness jocks, and other men can and do become obsessed with having the perfect body. These men will go to extremes to achieve the ideal weight and appearance: taking steroids, working out several hours a day, bingeing and purging.

In mixed gender groups focusing on food and body connections, issues of both men and women need to be taken into account, so that common problems are identified while differences are recognized and addressed. For simplicity—and because the vast majority of women have significant issues with food and body connections—feminine pronouns are used throughout this book. Substitute gender neutral terms as needed for your audience.

Anyone struggling with food or body conflicts needs support. When these issues are explored in a safe, respectful group environment, the opportunities for growth, understanding, and healing are enhanced. Groups have the potential to reduce feelings of isolation, build feelings of connection and interdependence, challenge narrow thinking, encourage risk-taking, and support people in making positive life changes.

The exercises in this book are intended for use in the context of some ongoing group, program, or support system on which the participant can depend over some length of time. Because this is so important, each exercise includes suggestions for how to adapt the process for ongoing groups.

But groups are not for everyone, so many of our exercises can also be adapted for individual use. For suggestions about which exercises are appropriate for individuals, refer to the **Visual Guide to Exercises** (p. xv) or create your own adaptation suited to the needs of your clients, patients, or students.

OTHER CONSIDERATIONS AND CAUTIONS

Know yourself. Be aware of your own attitudes, beliefs, and behaviors in rela-tion to food and body. Take the **What's My Focus?** behavior assessment (p. 124) and try the **Fat Attitudes** exercise (p. 131) with trusted friends or colleagues. Write your own **Past Connections** (p. 115) to describe your personal history with food and weight conflicts. The more homework you do to understand yourself and to raise your consciousness about the complexity of food and weight problems or the painful effects of size discrimination, the greater your chances of being helpful to others.

Know your audience. Think about the potential composition of your group. What do you know about participants' educational background, occupational group, marital status, sexual orientation, age, gender, socioeconomic level, cultural diversity, ethnic values, traditions, and lifestyle? Is your audience familiar with the type of material or group processes you will be presenting, or will your ideas be brand new or scary for people? Is the material appropriate for the setting and audience? Is the level of disclosure appropriate? What questions do you antici-pate? What resources do you think are needed? What kinds of problems do you think they might have with food, body image, and overall health? The better you know your audience, the greater your chances of making your session pertinent to their needs. Check the **Visual Guide to Exercises** for guidelines.

Know the medical realities. While this book is biased toward non-dieting approaches to eating, many people do have weight-related medical conditions—such as diabetes—that require restrictive diets and/or controlled eating. Remember that these people are likely to be in your audience and their special needs should be acknowledged. Under no circumstances should they be encouraged to participate in activities that could endanger their physical health or undermine their ongoing medical care. *Self-acceptance is not the same as complacency*—or irresponsibility. Encourage participants to accept their medical conditions and care for themselves wisely.

Know your material. Use your own professional library and other available resources to read widely about the topic. Check the bibliography in the Resources section (p. 176) for reading suggestions. Study current research about effects of dieting on body weight, gender differences in body image, and other relevant topics. Talk to other professionals about their experiences, or organize a focus group of professionals (educators, trainers, support group leaders, and therapists) in your community who are working in these areas of health. Listen to participants themselves talk about their experiences, successes, and failures. Learn from them.

Know your resources. Find out what is available locally. Talk to program directors, support group leaders, physicians, nutritionists, dietitians, therapists, and educators about their classes, programs, groups, or other resources. Learn about their credentials, professional theories, and attitudes. Gather specific information about program location, cost, screening procedures, times of meetings, phone numbers, and names of contact persons. Investigate state and national resources: organizations such as the National Center for Overcoming Overeating and the National Association to Advance Fat Acceptance (NAAFA); magazines, newsletters, and journals; and video and audiotapes available on the topic. *Always bring local resource lists for participants* of any new workshop or group session and make sure that every participant gets one.

Know when and how to set group boundaries. Think ahead about what is appropriate disclosure for your group. Make sure that participants understand what is going to happen in the group process, and advocate for their right to say no to any activity that makes them uncomfortable or violates their personal boundaries. Protect all participants from inappropriate disclosures by making group purpose, limits, and expectations as clear as possible. Rehearse how you will handle inappropriate disclosures, emotional responses, or other challenging events that may occur during the group process. Keep an alternative group activity in your back pocket for emergencies, in case you have to leave the room briefly to be with an emotional participant.

Know when and how to refer. Decide on clear criteria for group participation. If you are doing a workplace wellness presentation, it is not necessary to do a pregroup screening or require a medical examination. The same principles apply to onetime community education workshops.

In the screening process and during the course of your group or educational process, be alert for possible eating disorders. Become familiar with the typical symptoms of eating disorders (eg, distorted body image, clothing as camouflage, over exercising, bingeing, vomiting, secrecy and denial about eating patterns, self-abusive language, etc). When you suspect an applicant or participant may have an active eating disorder, refer her to the appropriate resources in your community for evaluation and treatment. This is when the background work you did on community resources will pay off. Facilitate the referral in whatever way you can, support the person through the process, and provide appropriate follow-up.

HOW TO USE THIS BOOK

The 36 exercises in this book are designed to involve participants creatively in the learning process, regardless of setting or time constraints. To aid you in the selection of appropriate exercises, they are grouped into five broad categories:

◆ **Icebreakers:** These short, engaging exercises are designed to help participants warm up to the topic and to each other. Try combining an icebreaker with one of the main focus exercises for a ready-made program session.

◆ **Focus on Food and Eating Issues:** These exercises include practical, powerful processes for exploring each person's relationship with food. There are exercises focused on social/cultural, emotional, spiritual, mental, physical, and sensory factors influencing hunger and eating, along with a variety of ideas for how participants might break out of unhealthy patterns and develop flexible, balanced, holistic ways to nourish themselves.

◆ **Focus on Body Image and Movement:** Exercises in this section will help participants explore personal body image from many perspectives: enjoyable movement, positive and negative attitudes and beliefs about body, historical roots of these body beliefs, and deeper connections to the inner self.

◆ **Focus on Attitudes: Cultural and Personal:** These exercises challenge participants to look at their own attitudes about food and eating, body size, appearance, dieting, beauty, fat people, and overall definitions of health—from both a personal and a cultural perspective. They are designed to stimulate thinking, raise consciousness, and stretch participants' (and trainers') attitudes from traditional views of weight and body size to new attitudes that are based on increased respect for diversity, including body size.

◆ **Group Energizers:** All groups need a change of pace—a process for taking a breather, for refueling mentally or physically and returning to the group session with renewed energy. The energizers in this section include a rich selection: some with food and eating as a nourishing and educational break, some that use the imagination to alter attitudes toward eating, and others with physical activity as an action-oriented way to get energized.

The format is designed for easy use. You'll find that each exercise is described completely, including: goals, group size, time frame, materials needed, step-by-step process instructions, and applications for use with ongoing groups. Graphic symbols are used throughout to indicate the type of process:

☞ *The hand points to helpful hints and special instructions for the presenter.*

● Chalktalk (mini-lecture) points are designated by a bullet.

✔ Questions for large group input, brainstorming, or discussion are preceded by a check.

➤ Step-by-step directions for group activities are indicated by an arrow.

Scripts to be read to the group are typed in italics.

At the end of this book you will find a resource section listing related books, magazines, newsletters, journals, organizations, videotapes, and audiocassettes. This list is by no means comprehensive, but it offers a solid core of suggestions for your professional library or resource network. Information about the twenty-five contributors to this volume are also included in this section.

VISUAL GUIDE TO EXERCISES

To assist you in choosing appropriate exercises for your group and setting, we have included a **Visual Guide to Exercises** that categorizes the exercises by exercise number, page, title, time frame, appropriate settings (workplace wellness, community education, weight management programs, ongoing growth/support groups, therapy groups, or professional education groups), and appropriate target audiences (general public, people with diet-sensitive medical problems, women only, or individuals).

The **Visual Guide** also indicates the type of process used, the level of participant disclosure required, the level of trainer preparation, and the need for scripts, worksheets, A-V equipment, and other materials.

KEY TO THE VISUAL GUIDE

Materials: A ✂ indicates the need for extra materials such as art supplies, reference books, or other supplies noted in the exercise.

Worksheets: A ✎ symbolizes that worksheets are necessary for participant reflection.

Script: A ❞ notes that the exercise includes a script to be read by the trainer. This may be a guided image, story, parable, or set of instructions.

Smallgroup: A ❖ indicates that the exercise includes small group (2–6 persons) process or interaction.

Disclosure: Different levels of disclosure are appropriate with different audiences and settings.

Blank = No significant self-disclosure.
- ❶ = Brief/Low-level sharing in response to open-ended questions of non-sensitive nature. Each individual chooses how much to disclose.
- ❷ = Personal sharing in response to direct questions about somewhat sensitive issues. Opportunity for disclosure of current strengths/problems. Feedback/affirmation.
- ❸ = Opportunity for deeper disclosure about potentially painful subjects. Pointed questions/assessment.

Trainer Preparation: This includes the gathering of necessary materials as well as the experience of the leader.

Blank = No preparation time needed, ready to go as is.
- ❶ = Easy, but needs materials and/or preparation.
- ❷ = Some preparation needed; content/process suitable to most trainers.
- ❸ = Longer/more complicated exercise; requires extensive preparation and/or sophisticated judgment by trainer.

VISUAL GUIDE TO EXERCISES

Exercise	Page	TITLE	Time (minutes)	Worksheets	Script	Materials	A-V Materials	(Editor's) Favorites
ICEBREAKERS								
1	2	What Kind of Food Am I?	5–10					☆
2	3	It's My Body	5–15			✄		☆
3	5	Pyramid	10–15	✎		✄		
4	9	As I See It	15–20	✎		✄		
5	12	Diets I've Known	15–20	✎		✄		
6	15	My Problem Is . . .	10–15					
7	17	Work of Art	10–15			✄		☆
FOCUS on: FOOD & EATING ISSUES								
8	22	Easy as Pie?	25–30	✎				
9	29	Influencing Factors	45–60	✎				
10	36	Clean Plate Club	30–45	✎		✄		
11	44	Sensational Diet	60–90	✎		✄		☆
12	50	Food House Fantasy	45–60	✎	99			☆
13	57	Spiritual Hunger	60–90	✎	99	✄		☆
14	62	Food: The Feeling Plug	30–40	✎				
15	68	Whole Person Snack Pack	45–60	✎			●	
16	74	Ideal Patterns	45–60					
FOCUS on: BODY IMAGE & MOVEMENT								
17	82	Body Parts	30–40	✎		✄		☆
18	87	Finding Center	20–30		99	✄	●	
19	92	Mirror, Mirror	30–45	✎		✄		☆

	Appropriate Setting							Audience				Process	
	Workplace Wellness	Community Education	Weight Mgmt Programs	Ongoing Growth/Support Groups	Therapy Groups	Professional Education Groups	General Public	Diet-Sensitive Medical Problems	Women Only	Individuals	Small Groups	Disclosure	Trainer Preparation
ICEBREAKERS													
	●	●	●	●	●	●	●	●			●		
			●	●	●	●		●			●	❷	❶
	●	●	●	●		●	●	●			●	❷	❷
	●	●	●	●	●	●	●	●			●	❶	❶
	●	●	●	●	●	●		●			●	❷	❷
		●	●	●	●	●	●		●	●	●	❷	
				●	●	●	●		●		●	❷	❷
FOCUS on: FOOD & EATING ISSUES													
	●	●	●	●	●	●	●	●		●	●	❷	❷
	●	●	●	●	●	●	●	●		●		❷	❷
	●	●	●	●	●	●	●	●		●	●	❷	❷
		●	●	●		●		●			●	❶	❸
		●		●	●	●				●	●	❷	❷
			●	●	●	●				●	●	❷	❷
	●	●	●	●	●	●	●	●		●	●	❷	❷
	●	●		●	●		●	●		●		❶	❷
	●	●	●	●	●	●	●	●					❶
FOCUS on: BODY IMAGE & MOVEMENT													
	●	●	●	●	●	●	●	●		●	●	❷	❷
	●	●	●	●	●	●	●	●		●	●	❶	❶
		●		●	●			●		●		❷	❷

VISUAL GUIDE TO EXERCISES

Exercise	Page	TITLE	Time (minutes)	Worksheets	Script	Materials	A-V Materials	(Editor's) Favorites
20	99	Moving Attitudes	45	✎				☆
21	106	Physical Activity Continuum	45–60			✂		☆
22	110	Sensual Walk	20–30					
23	115	Past Connections	40–50	✎	99	✂		
FOCUS on: ATTITUDES: CULTURAL & PERSONAL								
24	124	What's My Focus?	25–30	✎				☆
25	131	Fat Attitudes	45–60		99	✂	●	☆
26	136	Myths and Realities	45–60	✎		✂		
27	144	Beauty Chant	15–20		99		●	☆
28	148	Fat Chance	15–20	✎		✂		☆
29	153	Who Says So?	10–20			✂	●	
GROUP ENERGIZERS								
30	158	Pleasant Thoughts	5–10			✂		
31	160	Body Count	5–10					
32	162	Fans of Mozart	5–10			✂	●	
33	164	Fight Song	10–15		99			
34	166	Snack Cafeteria	20			✂		
35	169	Mindful Eating Experience	5–15			✂		☆
36	172	Empty Calories	5–10		99			

	Appropriate Setting						Audience					Process	
	Workplace Wellness	Community Education	Weight Mgmt Programs	Ongoing Growth/Support Groups	Therapy Groups	Professional Education Groups	General Public	Diet-Sensitive Medical Problems	Women Only	Individuals	Small Groups	Disclosure	Trainer Preparation
				●	●	●						❷	❸
	●	●	●			●	●	●			●	❷	❶
	●	●	●	●		●	●	●				❶	❶
			●	●	●	●		●		●	●	❸	❷
FOCUS on: ATTITUDES: CULTURAL & PERSONAL													
	●	●	●	●	●	●	●	●		●		❷	❷
		●		●		●	●	●				❷	❸
		●		●		●	●				●	❶	❷
		●		●			●		●		●	❶	❶
		●	●	●			●				●	❷	❶
		●		●	●		●	●			●	❷	❷
GROUP ENERGIZERS													
	●	●	●	●	●	●	●	●		●		❶	❶
	●	●	●	●		●	●	●		●			
	●	●	●	●		●	●	●					❶
		●	●	●		●	●				●		❶
	●	●	●	●		●	●	●			●		❸
	●	●	●	●	●	●	●	●		●	●		❶
	●	●	●	●		●	●	●					

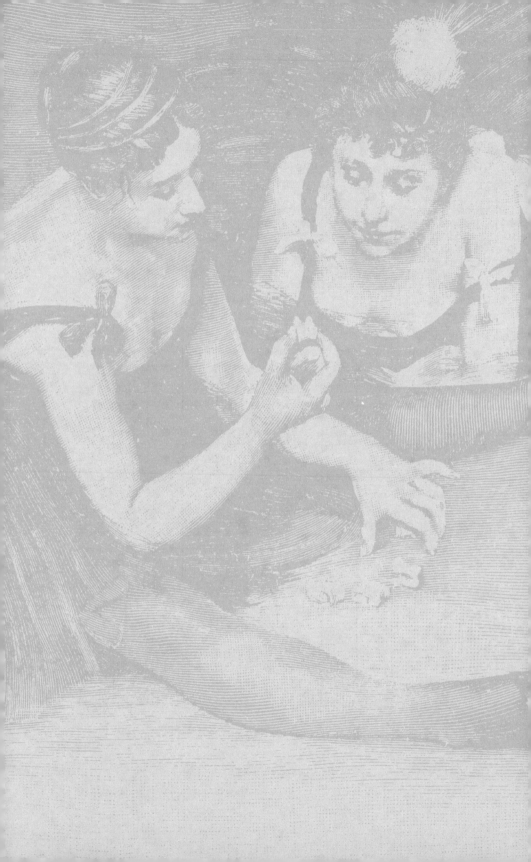

ICEBREAKERS

These short, engaging exercises are designed to help participants warm up to the topic—and to each other. Try combining an icebreaker with one of the main focus exercises for a ready-made program session.

1   WHAT KIND OF FOOD AM I?   page 2
Participants use a food metaphor to describe their personality and introduce themselves. (5–10 min.)

2   IT'S MY BODY   page 3
Participants sculpt a paper cup to describe feelings about their bodies and use their creations for introductions. (5–15 min.)

3   PYRAMID   page 5
In this unique mixer, participants get acquainted by sharing stories about the degree to which their daily food choices match dietary guidelines of the food pyramid. (10–15 min.)

4   AS I SEE IT   page 9
In this engaging icebreaker, participants heighten awareness of personal values and attitudes about health and wellness. (15–20 min.)

5   DIETS I'VE KNOWN   page 12
This engaging icebreaker will give participants an opportunity to talk about their dieting history in an open, accepting environment. (15–20 min.)

6   MY PROBLEM IS . . .   page 15
This simple, subjective assessment focuses on what is bothering participants about relationships with food and body. (10–15 min.)

7   WORK OF ART   page 17
Women participants use reproductions of museum masterpieces to discover a work of art that represents their own beauty, creativity, and uniqueness. (10–15 min.)

1 WHAT KIND OF FOOD AM I?

Participants use a food metaphor to describe their personality and introduce themselves.

GOALS

To get acquainted with other participants.

To warm up to the subject matter of the session.

GROUP SIZE

Unlimited. Works best with groups of 8–10, but several groups can participate simultaneously.

TIME FRAME

5–10 minutes.

PROCESS

1. Start with a metaphorical question.

   ✔ What type of food would best describe your personality?

   ☞ *Give examples to stimulate ideas: Are you like a potato, salt of the earth with many "eyes" for perception? Or like a loaf of bread, soft, warm, and filling? Or an enchilada, hot and spicy?*

2. After participants have had a chance to think of an appropriate food, ask everyone to use this food metaphor as an introduction.

   ➤ Introduce yourself to the group by stating your name, the type of food that represents your personality, and a brief explanation of why you picked that particular food.

© 1996 WHOLE PERSON PRESS 210 WEST MICHIGAN DULUTH MN 55802 ■ (800) 247-6789

2 IT'S MY BODY

Participants sculpt a paper cup to describe feelings about their bodies and use their creations for introductions.

GOALS

To make introductions.

To get in touch with body image issues.

GROUP SIZE

Unlimited. Works best with groups of 8–10, but several groups can participate simultaneously.

TIME FRAME

5–15 minutes.

MATERIALS NEEDED

Paper or Styrofoam cup for each participant.

PROCESS

1. Ask participants to sit in a circle and give everyone a Styrofoam or paper cup.

2. Give instructions for the first round of introductions.

   ➤ The cup is a metaphor for how you feel about your body. One by one introduce yourself to the group, using your cup as a symbolic way of showing the group how you feel about your body.

   ➤ When it is your turn to introduce yourself, pick up the cup, and *without talking,* do something with the cup that symbolizes your feelings about your body.

      ➤ You can do whatever you want with the cup, as long as you do it nonverbally.

      ➤ Be brief (10–15 seconds per person).

3. When all have introduced themselves nonverbally, give instructions for verbal introductions.

   ➤ Go around the group again, introducing yourself by name and briefly explain why you chose the symbolic actions you did.

© 1996 WHOLE PERSON PRESS 210 WEST MICHIGAN DULUTH MN 55802 ■(800) 247-6789

4. When the second go-around is completed, summarize the diversity of feelings that participants have about their bodies and reassure everyone that all feelings—positive, mixed, and negative—are accepted. Then move on to your next agenda, weaving in body image issues if appropriate.

FOR ONGOING GROUPS

■ This metaphor can be used to represent other issues, relationships, or feelings of participants. It can be a powerful lead-in for whatever topic your group is exploring.

3 PYRAMID

In this unique mixer, participants get acquainted by sharing stories about the degree to which their daily food choices match dietary guidelines of the food pyramid.

GOALS

To get acquainted.

To learn about the food pyramid as a guide to daily food choices.

GROUP SIZE

Unlimited.

TIME FRAME

10–15 minutes.

MATERIALS NEEDED

Food Pyramid handouts; six large posters, prepared in advance by the trainer, representing each food group of the food pyramid and labeled to correspond to each food group on the pyramid handout. Display these posters at six different locations around the room.

PROCESS

☞ *The food pyramid guide used here was developed by the United States Department of Agriculture and Health and Human Services. If you live elsewhere, adapt the handout and presentation to your national nutrition guidelines.*

1. Introduce the food pyramid by explaining that it is a model of dietary guidelines for daily food choices developed by the United States Department of Agriculture and Health and Human Services. Distribute copies of the **Food Pyramid** handout and give a brief presentation about the pyramid model.

2. Invite participants to reflect on the extent to which their own daily food choices match the dietary guidelines of the pyramid model, and then use these reflections as an opportunity for getting to know other participants.

   ➤ Look over the food pyramid and the recommended daily servings for each food category.

➤ Considering your typical eating habits, which food group do you need to eat *more* of?

➤ Notice that there are posters placed around the room for each food category of the pyramid. Find the poster of the food group that you need to eat *more* of, then go to that location.

➤ When you get to your chosen food group, pair up with another participant at that food category station and exchange ideas about changing your eating habits in this category.

➤ Each person has 2 minutes to share your dietary needs and ideas.

3. Interrupt the small group discussions and invite participants to explore another aspect of their daily food choices.

➤ Think again about the food pyramid and the recommended number of servings for each food group.

➤ Considering your typical eating habits, which food group do you need to eat *less* of?

➤ Find the location of that food group and go to that spot.

➤ Pair up with another participant and discuss how you might change your eating patterns related to this food group.

➤ Each person has 2 minutes to share your dietary needs and ideas.

4. Interrupt the group discussions again and give instructions for the final round of sharing.

➤ Continue to use the food pyramid as a guide for reflection.

➤ What food group do you think you eat in *just about the right amounts?*

➤ Find the location for this food group and go to that spot in the room.

➤ Pair up with another participant in this food group and exchange stories about foods you eat that match the recommendations of the food pyramid.

➤ Each person has 2 minutes to share whatever you like about how you succeed in following these dietary guidelines.

5. Reconvene the group and ask participants to share examples of insights, commonalties discovered, questions or concerns raised. Use this discussion as a launchpad for more in-depth teaching about the food pyramid or for moving on to your next group agenda.

FOR ONGOING GROUPS

▓ For an interesting and fun application of the pyramid model to daily food choices, adapt Exercise 34, **Snack Cafeteria** (p. 166) to the food pyramid guide. Prepare portions of various foods from all pyramid groups in the cafeteria offerings.

Use miniature cards cut into shapes representing each food group of the pyramid and label them accordingly. On the menu, include the recommended number of servings for each food group.

Set the pyramid pieces out in a stack beside the appropriate foods in the cafeteria line and have participants take a corresponding shape for each food they choose, so they will have visual tokens for all the foods they selected. When they sit down, they can try to put their pyramid together, like a puzzle, and thereby learn what food is over-represented or underrepresented in their diet.

Contributed by Nancy Loving Tubesing.

© 1996 WHOLE PERSON PRESS 210 WEST MICHIGAN DULUTH MN 55802 ■ (800) 247-6789

FOOD PYRAMID

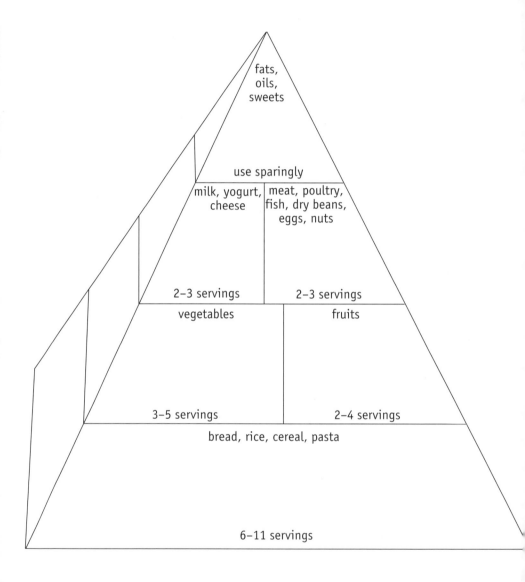

4 AS I SEE IT

In this engaging icebreaker, participants heighten awareness of personal values and attitudes about health and wellness.

GOALS

To promote self-awareness about values and attitudes affecting personal health care choices.

To get acquainted.

GROUP SIZE

Works best with groups of 20 or more. With fewer participants, use a progression of small groups (2s, 4s, 8s, or 3s, 6s) instead of the mixer.

TIME FRAME

15–20 minutes.

MATERIALS NEEDED

As I See It worksheets; whistle, horn, or harmonica to signal time to change partners.

PROCESS

1. Distribute **As I See It** worksheets and invite participants to express, in writing, their attitudes about wellness.

   ➤ Complete each of the eight sentences with whatever thoughts come to your mind. Work quickly.

2. When everyone has finished the worksheet (allow 3–5 minutes), give instructions for the mixer.

   ☞ *Demonstrate the sound cue you will use to get the group's attention.*

   ➤ Stand up, move around the room, find a partner, then introduce yourself.

   ➤ Take turns reading your **first sentence** *(I think wellness means . . .)* and briefly explain your response to it.

   ➤ Each pair has 1 minute to exchange answers.

   ➤ When the whistle blows, move on to a new person and talk about your response to the **second sentence** *(I think illness means . . .).*

➤ Each time the whistle blows, find a new partner and answer the next question on your list, until all eight have been answered.

☞ *If you are planning to use small groups in your next agenda component, instruct pairs to form quartets (or sextets) for the last round of sentence sharing.*

3. Solicit examples from participants about sentence completions they found most intriguing or relevant. If possible, connect comments with the purpose, agenda, and philosophy of your group.

4. Conclude with a chalktalk about the connection between values, attitudes, and health care choices.

● **Values and attitudes are at the core of all the choices we make** about self-care. If you value thinness more than personal vitality, you might sacrifice nutrition by skipping meals or chronic dieting. If your attitude toward yourself is accepting and respectful, you are more likely to take good care of yourself. If you think health care professionals cannot help you, you are less likely to seek help for any health concern, including weight and eating issues.

● **Be aware of your attitudes and values.** Give yourself periodic checkups to see if your lifestyle is in line with your attitudes and values. If not, ask yourself what needs adjustment to restore balance between what you believe and how you live.

FOR ONGOING GROUPS

▓ Rewrite the sentences to suit the special concerns or issues of your group. Create sentence stems for topics such as eating disorders, body image, dieting, self-esteem, or exercise, then invite group members to go around and share one or more sentences as a lead-in to these topics.

Contributed by Sandy Queen.

© 1996 WHOLE PERSON PRESS 210 WEST MICHIGAN DULUTH MN 55802 ■(800) 247-6789

AS I SEE IT

I think wellness means . . .

I think illness means . . .

I feel well when . . .

I feel not so well when . . .

Some people can be healthy but not well because . . .

I think people who are out of shape are . . .

I think food contributes to wellness by . . .

Doctors and health professionals can . . .

5 DIETS I'VE KNOWN

This engaging icebreaker will give participants an opportunity to talk about their dieting history in an open, accepting environment.

GOALS

To get acquainted.

To affirm the efforts of all participants who have suffered on diets.

GROUP SIZE

Unlimited.

TIME FRAME

15–20 minutes.

MATERIALS NEEDED

Diets I've Known worksheets; newsprint and marker; 5–6 *Badge of Courage* buttons for winners of the *most outrageous diet contest;* affirmation stickers (blue ribbons, positive messages, etc) for all participants.

PROCESS

1. Start with an intriguing definition of dieting from the *Feminist Dictionary.*

   ● **Dieting involves weight watching and appetite-controlling techniques** directed primarily at women and designed to reduce the body, make it smaller, narrow, lightweight, lose gravity, belittle, shrink, confine, contract, lessen. The emphasis is on restraint and prohibition, on confining and controlling hungers.

2. Invite participants to brainstorm a list of all the diets they've tried, including exercise programs and other methods of losing weight. Use newsprint to record all ideas generated.

   ☞ *As participants identify weight-loss strategies, ask a few to share details about particularly intriguing diets. If necessary, prime the pump with suggestions (eg, Scarsdale, Weight Watchers, grapefruit and egg, Nutra-System, Diet Center, Weight Loss Clinic, diet pills, laxatives, low-fat diet, high-protein diet, etc).*

3. Observe that there are over 30,000 diet plans in America so it is no surprise that many people have tried several of them. Hand out **Diets I've Known** worksheets and ask participants to reflect on their personal diet history.

➤ On the left side of the measuring cup, in the column labeled **Diets,** list all the diets you've tried in your lifetime including exercise programs.

➣ List as many as you can in 1 minute.

➣ If your list is too long for the space, let the diets spill over the top of the cup and down the side of the page.

➤ Estimate the *number of pounds you lost* and the *money you spent* on each diet. Record these numbers in the appropriate columns and add the **Totals**.

4. Give instructions for forming groups and guidelines for sharing.

➤ Find two or three people who have also tried one of the diets on your list.

➣ No more than four in a group.

➤ Place your chairs in a circle.

➤ Go around the group and introduce yourselves.

➤ Take 2 minutes each to talk about some of the diets you've tried and describe how you felt to be on them.

➣ The person with the least full measuring cup serves as the timekeeper.

5. When everyone has had time to share their stories, invite participants to share examples of the *most outrageous diets* they talked about in their group.

6. Ask participants to vote on the *most outrageous diet* and give *Badge of Courage* awards to all participants who tried this diet. Give all participants affirmative stickers for their courage, persistence, and determination.

7. In closing, remind participants never to blame themselves for the failure of a diet: research shows that diets are a proven failure as a method of permanent weight loss.

● **Diets don't work.** Studies have shown that frequent dieting increases the likelihood of lowering your metabolism; slowing weight loss; becoming hypersensitive to food cues; developing a pattern of overeating, bingeing, or bulimia. Yo-yo dieters tend to regain weight three times more quickly than they lost it. These failures belong to the *diet,* not the *dieter.*

Adapted from a presentation led by Laura Field at a National Wellness conference. Laura credits Geneen Roth for the original idea.

DIETS I'VE KNOWN

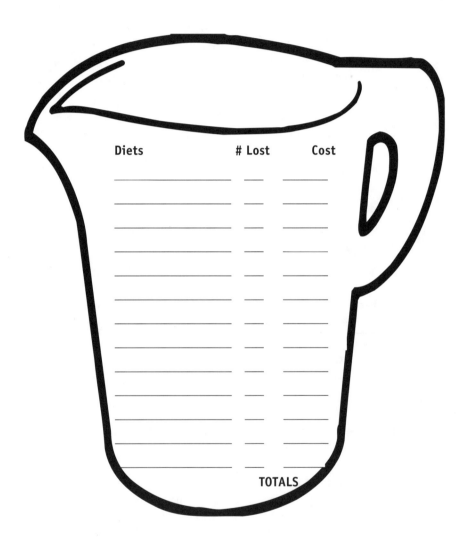

Diets	# Lost	Cost
	TOTALS	

6 MY PROBLEM IS . . .

This simple, subjective assessment focuses on what is bothering participants about relationships with food and body.

GOALS

To identify how these problems are causing pain or dis-ease and articulate personal problems with food or body.

To connect with other participants.

GROUP SIZE

Unlimited. Works best with groups of 10–12 participants, but can be done with several groups simultaneously.

TIME FRAME

10–15 minutes.

MATERIALS NEEDED

Blank sheets of paper.

PROCESS

1. After setting the tone for your learning experience, invite participants to reflect on what brings them to the session. Distribute blank paper and give instructions for the self-assessment.

   ➤ Complete the sentence *My problem is . . .* with a description of your current issues with food, weight management, fitness, or body image.

      ➤ This should be an honest summary of why you are here. It can be something *you* see as a problem (eg, *I eat junk food all the time and can't stop*) or something *someone else* thinks is a problem (eg, *I have high blood pressure and my doctor says I have to lose weight*).

   ➤ Use up to 25 words to articulate your present concerns about food or body issues.

2. When everyone has finished writing, invite participants to share their problem statements with other participants.

   ➤ Introduce yourself by stating your name and reading your problem statement.

3. When introductions are finished, summarize the common problems and concerns of participants, incorporating these issues into an overview of your agenda for the session.

☞ *If several groups are making introductions simultaneously, solicit examples of problems from each group during this step.*

FOR ONGOING GROUPS

▨ Ask participants to save their problem statements (eg, copy them into an ongoing journal). Repeat this exercise several sessions later to explore how people's perceptions of their problems have changed. Invite comments on how the group experience has influenced problem statements.

© 1996 WHOLE PERSON PRESS 210 WEST MICHIGAN DULUTH MN 55802 ■(800) 247-6789

7 WORK OF ART

Women participants use reproductions of museum masterpieces to discover a work of art that represents their own beauty, creativity, and uniqueness.

GOALS

To discover and affirm personal images of beauty that promote a positive body image.

To get acquainted.

GROUP SIZE

Unlimited. Works best with small groups, but several groups can work simultaneously, provided the trainer has enough art prints/postcards.

TIME FRAME

10-15 minutes.

MATERIALS NEEDED

Fine art postcards or prints of paintings, posters, photographs, or sculptures featuring women of different sizes, ages, and moods: one per participant, with several extras. Postcard books of women in art are available in the gift shops of many museums or directly from Whole Person Associates, 210 West Michigan Street, Duluth MN 55802, 800-247-6789. Newsprint posters indicating small group names and meeting locations.

PROCESS

☞ *Be sure you have 4–6 more prints/postcards than expected participants. Before the session, determine how many groups of 8–10 you expect in your audience. Use Post-it notes to label the backside of each postcard/ print with a number or name to signify group assignments (eg, by colors, by medium, or by schools of art).*

1. Before participants arrive, pin postcards/prints on the wall or spread them on a table at the back of the room where they will be inconspicuous but easily accessible.

2. Welcome participants and explain that as a way of getting acquainted participants will visit a miniature art museum and find a work of art they identify with. Give instructions.

➤ In the back of the room is a space representing a miniature art museum. On the table (or wall) are reproductions of famous paintings and sculptures from many different artists and time periods.

➤ You are invited to visit the museum, look at the gallery of art, and choose one work of art that you identify with—one that best depicts your unique beauty, body style, creativity, spirit, or soul.

➤ You may be attracted to several works of art—choose any one that seems to have some connection for you.

➤ Once you've made your selection, turn the artwork over and find your group assignment on the Post-it note. Go to that area of the room and wait for the rest of your group to gather.

➤ Do not reveal your work of art until it's time for your introduction.

3. When all participants have selected a work of art from the museum collection and have joined their small groups, give directions for introductions.

➤ The person who selected the oldest masterpiece goes first. Check the date on your card to determine when your work of art was created.

➤ Introduce yourself to the group by taking on the identity of your work of art.

➤ State your name.

➤ Complete the sentence:
I am a work of art by (artist) because . . .

➤ State all of the ways you are like this image or how you identify with it (eg, body type, beauty, mood, creativity, etc).

➤ Only positive, affirming statements are allowed. No sarcastic, ridiculing, or hostile put-downs of yourself, nor jokes that might belittle your appearance or personality.

4. When participants have finished introducing themselves, encourage everyone to continue thinking of themselves as a work of art with many unique and beautiful features. Suggest that participants visit an art museum and look for additional images in art that will affirm their body size, beauty, and creativity.

© 1996 WHOLE PERSON PRESS 210 WEST MICHIGAN DULUTH MN 55802 ■ (800) 247-6789

FOR ONGOING GROUPS

■ Expand this introduction with another sentence completion in *Step 4: If an artist were to paint me today, or create an image that would immortalize my beauty, she would create a work of art that looked like . . .*

■ Have each participant create her own work of art to celebrate her body and spirit.

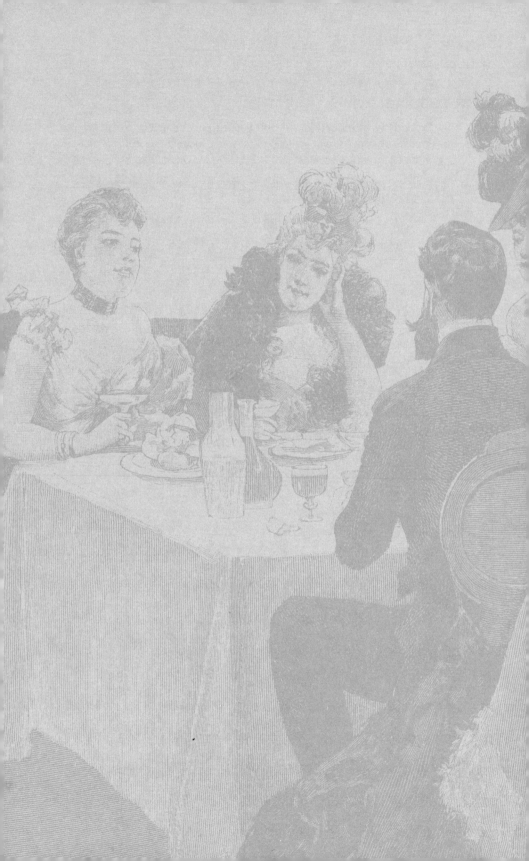

FOCUS ON
FOOD & EATING ISSUES

These exercises include practical and powerful processes for exploring relationships with food. The exercises focus on social/cultural, emotional, spiritual, mental, physical, and sensory factors that influence hunger and eating. They also provide a variety of ideas that help participants break out of unhealthy patterns and develop flexible, balanced, holistic ways to nourish themselves.

8 EASY AS PIE?

Participants who want to lose weight for health reasons use a pie chart to analyze components of their weight problem, then explore practical, commonsense choices for losing weight.

GOALS

To develop an understanding of personal weight problems.

To explore possibilities for losing weight in a healthy way and to develop an individualized plan for change.

GROUP SIZE

Unlimited.

TIME FRAME

25–30 minutes.

MATERIALS NEEDED

Easy as Pie? worksheets; newsprint, marker, and masking tape.

PROCESS

1. Start with a short chalktalk about the ease of gaining weight and the difficulty of losing it.

   ● **Gaining weight is as easy as pie.** Ask anyone who has struggled with this problem and they will tell you how easy it is to gain 10, 20, or even 30 pounds in a short period of time. Vacations, new jobs, pregnancy, stress, change of lifestyle (from active to sedentary), holidays, repeated dieting, and many other factors can cause you to gain weight quickly.

   ● **Losing weight is tough.** There is no quick, easy way to lose weight. Diets may produce rapid, temporary weight loss, but the pounds come back as soon as you start to eat normally again. Most experts agree that the only way to lose weight and keep it off is to make slow, gradual changes in your eating habits and lifestyle.

   ● **Most people can lose some weight.** How much weight can be lost will vary from individual to individual, depending on personal set-point, heredity, lifestyle, and the particular components of your weight problem. If most of your weight problem is due to overeating, and you find a way to change this pattern, your chances of returning to your natural (not ideal) body weight are quite good. Even a relatively small weight loss of 10 pounds can yield significant health benefits, so don't let *all or nothing thinking* stop you from valuing small changes.

2. Distribute **Easy As Pie?** worksheets and ask participants to write their problem statements on the back.

   ➤ What is your *reason* for wanting to lose weight?

   ➤ What is your *weight loss goal* (number of pounds, time period, maintenance)?

3. Invite participants to share personal reasons for wanting to lose weight, and list these motivations on newsprint. Encourage participants to find additional reasons beyond those based on appearance or pleasing others, since these externally-focused motivations have little to do with personal health and are unlikely to be helpful in making long-term change.

   ☞ *Solicit a wide variety of reasons, including:* **medical** *(need surgery, diabetes, high cholesterol, hypertension, heart disease);* **physical** *(joints hurt, back pain, lack of flexibility, strength, or endurance);* **social** *(can't keep up with the kids, limits my movement, restricts lifestyle, stops me from doing what I want to do);* **mental/psychological** *(want to practice better self-care, be healthier, change self-defeating behavior, improve self-esteem and confidence); and* **spiritual** *(want to experience personal growth through risk-taking, letting go, experiencing feelings in a new way without emotional eating).*

4. Summarize and affirm participants' reasons for wanting to lose weight, pointing out the wide variety of motivations in the group.

   Then invite participants to reflect on the varied causes of their own weight problems as they listen to a chalktalk summarizing common behavior patterns that cause people to gain weight.

   ● There are at least **nine common, controllable behavior patterns that contribute to weight problems**. Making changes in any of these areas can positively affect your eating patterns—and help you lose weight and maintain your new weight.

   ● **Emotional eating.** When we eat in response to emotions, (boredom, anxiety, loneliness, anger) we are probably eating when we are not hungry. This means that you are taking in food that your body doesn't need, adding extra calories that, if not burned off, will cause weight gain. The more you use food as a tranquilizer, the greater your chances of gaining weight.

● **Overeating.** This is a lot like emotional eating: we take in food we don't need. We simply ignore, override, or miss our internal signals of fullness, perhaps because the food tastes so good, we don't want to stop. We all overeat sometimes, (Thanksgiving dinners, for example) and this is not a problem unless it becomes routine. When overeating is your usual pattern, your body adapts by storing excess calories as fat, and you are likely to gain weight.

● **Snacking.** Nutritious snacks eaten in moderation between meals can actually help you to lose weight because they keep your blood sugar level stable and make you less prone to overeating. But excessive snacking, even on nutritious foods, can lead to weight gain.

● **Food choices: lots of sugar and fat.** Everyone knows that these foods are loaded with calories and when eaten in excess, cause weight gain. Too much sugar can also wreak havoc with your blood sugar level, causing you to experience ups and downs in mood and energy. Too much fat forces your body to store the excess, resulting in higher weight and increased risk for heart disease and stroke.

● **Timing of eating.** Recent studies have shown that if you eat smaller, more frequent *daytime* meals you have a better chance of losing weight than if you eat big meals in the evening. This is because your metabolism slows down at night and calories are burned more slowly when you are sleeping. Skipping meals and then overloading at one or two meals is not helpful, regardless of time of day.

● **Social eating.** For some people, social eating is like a continual binge. The usual restraints fly out the window. We easily rationalize our indulgence by the social context: celebrations, parties, special meals with loved ones. All become occasions for abandoning caution. This pattern can become a lifestyle that affects weight.

● **Restaurant eating.** If you eat many of your meals in restaurants, you may be tempted to eat high fat, high calorie foods, or simply eat too much. Many restaurants give jumbo-sized portions: a typical serving of chicken (two breasts) contains nearly 12 ounces of protein—twice as much protein as you need. Eating out frequently can add unwanted pounds—easy as pie.

● **Deprivation/Splurge pattern.** Most people can relate to this pattern. We deprive ourselves for awhile, then let go of control and splurge. Usually we binge on the foods we have denied ourselves: chocolate, ice cream, cookies, and other *forbidden* foods. This pattern is so predictable that many experts now recommend that rather than completely eliminate these foods from your diet, you let yourself enjoy pleasure foods in a consistent, *moderate* way.

- **Exercise/Movement.** Exercise burns calories. If you are very sedentary, regular exercise is likely to help you lose weight and may also affect eating patterns in a healthy way. Experts recommend 20 minutes of aerobic activity (increasing your heart rate and sustaining it in a safe range for that time period) 5–6 times a week when you are trying to lose weight. Once you have reached your weight goal, exercising 3–4 times a week should maintain it.

5. Ask participants if they can think of any other common, controllable causes of weight gain that have not yet been mentioned. Then hand out **Easy as Pie?** worksheets and guide participants through an exploration of the components of their weight-problem pie.

   ➤ On the left side of the worksheet is a list of the **behaviors** that could be contributing to your weight problem. If there are other behaviors that you know cause you to gain weight or prevent you from losing it, add them to the list on your worksheet.

   ➤ The circle in the center represents your **weight problem.** Looking over the list of behaviors on the left, decide which ones contribute to your weight problem, and what portion/percentage of the pie they represent.

      ➤ Divide your weight problem pie into slices representing its components.

      ➤ Fill in all of your pie so that the total percentage equals 100%.

      ➤ Label each slice with the behavior it represents and its percentage.

6. When most participants have completed their problem pie, ask them to reconsider the appropriateness of their goal.

   ➤ Look over your pie, and think about the causes of your weight problem. When you reflect on these causes and your motivation to change your behavior, do your weight loss goals still seem reasonable?

7. Ask participants to share their discoveries and reflections with another group member.

   ➤ Pair up with another person you do not know well, and share what you have discovered about the pieces of your weight problem pie, as well as your thoughts about how reasonable or realistic you think your weight loss goals are.

   ➤ Each person has 2 minutes to share.

© 1996 WHOLE PERSON PRESS 210 WEST MICHIGAN DULUTH MN 55802 ■(800) 247-6789

8. Invite participants to share discoveries, reflections, concerns, or questions raised by completing the **Easy as Pie?** worksheets.

   ☞ *If any participants have started to have second thoughts about their weight loss goals, support their instinct to be cautious and encourage them to take all the time they need to evaluate information and decide what is best for them.*

9. Ask participants to brainstorm a list of possible strategies for each problem behavior category. Use a sheet of newsprint for each category, label it with the problem category being discussed, and hang all nine strategy lists along the wall or blackboard.

   Encourage participants to use their pie chart to take notes on strategies for the different components.

   ☞ *Come prepared with your own list of strategy suggestions for each problem component. For example:*

   Emotional eating: *express your feelings directly; use stress management.*

   Overeating: *slow down eating; use hunger scale.*

   Snacking: *substitute healthy snacks for sugary/high fat snacks; eat mid-morning and mid-afternoon snacks to sustain energy.*

   Food choices: *gradually wean off high fat/sugary foods; experiment with new foods and recipes.*

   Timing of eating: *never skip a meal, especially breakfast; eat several small meals throughout the day.*

   Social eating: *focus on the nonfood pleasures of socializing; eat before going to social events where you are likely to overeat.*

   Restaurant eating: *be assertive regarding how you want food prepared; put excess portions in a take-home container at the beginning of the meal.*

   Deprivation/Splurge: *never deprive yourself of food; don't skip meals, diet, or fast; allow yourself to eat some favorite food in moderation.*

   Exercise/Movement: *start with small changes; build up to more challenging movement; find exercise that you enjoy.*

10. Guide participants in further reflection about healthy options for losing weight.

    ➤ Consider the components of your weight problem as well as your current life situation, values, lifestyle, and motivation for losing weight.

➤ Given all these factors, how can you lose weight without becoming obsessed about it?

➢ Identify several behaviors or strategies that are likely to help you change one or more pieces of the pie.

➢ Make a list of your best options for change in the top part of the **Best Choices for Change** column on your worksheet.

➤ Now look over the list and decide what you *will* change and what you *won't* change.

➢ Write what you *will change* in the space labeled, **I will** (eg, *give up my bedtime snack of peanuts, meditate for 20 minutes instead*).

➢ Write what you *won't change* in the space labeled **I won't** (eg, *go on another diet, give up candy bars*) on your worksheet.

11. Solicit examples from participants of their plans for change and then wrap up with practical suggestions for applying strategies to weight loss goals.

● **Take it slowly.** Any sudden change of diet, activity pattern, or lifestyle is going to challenge your body chemistry and your mind. Specific changes may provoke physiological and psychological resistances you don't want or need. Avoid this stress and frustration by giving yourself time to make slow, gradual, lasting changes in your eating and exercising habits. This will not upset the apple cart and will increase your chances of integrating and sustaining the changes you are trying to make.

FOR ONGOING GROUPS

▥ Focus on one or two strategies at a time, using time between group sessions to work on these changes and then using some scheduled group time to talk about progress.

▥ Develop a process for helping participants keep weight loss goals in perspective so they don't let weight loss become so important that they neglect other important areas of their lives. This could be a simple, subjective measure such a self-rated *preoccupation score* from 0–10, with *0* meaning *I never even **think** about losing weight* and *10* meaning *I think almost obsessively about losing weight.*

EASY AS PIE?

BEHAVIORS

Emotional eating

Overeating

Snacking

Food choices

Timing of eating

Social eating

Restaurant eating

Deprivation/Splurge patterns

Exercise/Movement

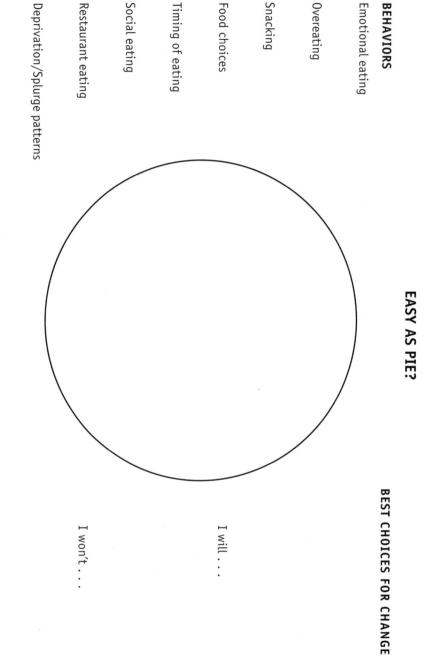

BEST CHOICES FOR CHANGE

I will . . . .

I won't . . . .

9 INFLUENCING FACTORS

Participants use an adaptation of a Japanese problem-solving technique to explore the multifaceted layers of their problems with food and weight.

GOALS

To appreciate the complexity of food and weight problems.
To identify specific factors influencing eating and body weight.
To identify goals and strategies for change.

GROUP SIZE

Unlimited. Also works well with individuals.

TIME FRAME

45–60 minutes.

MATERIALS NEEDED

Two copies of **Influencing Factors** worksheet for each participant; newsprint; marker.

PROCESS

1. Start by asking participants to brainstorm factors that might influence food and weight problems.

2. Incorporate responses into a short chalktalk about the complexity of food and weight problems.

   ● **Food and weight problems are complex.** Many factors influence our relationship with food and our bodies: genetics, diet or eating habits, physical activity, cultural values, social relationships, physical health and biological systems, emotional reactions to food, personal and family history, and other life variables such as illness, injury, age, stress, economics, and environment.

   ● **Understanding of food and weight problems is constantly changing.** It's hard to keep up with new information, let alone understand or trust it. Results of new scientific studies often contradict previous studies: butter is now considered healthier than margarine; maintaining a heavier, stable weight is better than dieting or experiencing chronic weight fluctuations.

● In the 1950s, appetite control through amphetamines was a common treatment for obesity; in the 1990s, set-point theory and the discovery of a gene linked to obesity have challenged thinking about dieting and weight problems. **There are differing perceptions of obesity:** is it a medical issue, a cultural issue, or a self-esteem issue? Who says it's a problem? There is no clear, simple answer to these questions.

3. Distribute **Influencing Factors** worksheets and explain that this is a visual model developed by dietitian Roxanne Bijold, RD, to help people understand the diverse factors influencing their food and weight problems.

4. Explain the worksheet and the process of reflection.
   ➤ This graphic presents a model of your food and weight problems. The nine sections represent the unfolding petals of a lotus blossom.
   ➤ The center of the blossom names the problem you are exploring today: food and weight problems.
   ➤ The eight outside petals represent unfolding factors that probably influence your food and weight problem.
      ➢ They are arranged alphabetically and unfold in a clockwise manner around the problem, from **A** to **I.**
      ➢ We will explore each factor in sequence, beginning with **A, Activity level.**

5. Lead a chalktalk and reflection process on each of the eight influencing factors.
   ● **A = Activity level.** The basic human metabolic equation is very simple. To maintain a specific weight, energy output must equal energy input. The calories taken in need to equal the calories burned. Increasing the activity level without increasing calorie intake should lead to weight loss over time.

   In real life, it's not quite so simple. Research suggests that the kind of calories (fat versus complex carbohydrates), as well as the timing of eating (bedtime versus midday) and/or exercising, may influence the metabolic equation substantially.
      ➢ How do you think your activity level affects your food and weight problem?
      ➢ In **Petal A,** write a couple of insights or examples of how *activity level* affects your food and weight problem.
   ● **B=Body type.** People come in all sizes and shapes. Each individual

is born with a unique body type and metabolism. This predisposition often affects body weight and appearance more than diet or exercise.

If you inherited a string bean body type and a very high metabolic rate, there is probably little you can do to gain weight or develop a soft, shapely body. Other women have pear-shaped bodies with fat deposits on their hips and thighs. While some women groan about having this body type, research has shown that it does put you at less risk for heart disease, diabetes, and stroke than a round apple shape with fat deposits in your abdominal area. However, people with all shapes can have food or weight problems.

➤ In what ways does your body type and metabolism influence your food and weight issues?

➤ Write your reflections about *body type* in **Petal B.**

● **C=Cultural/Social.** Many of us are influenced by the attitudes and values in our culture or social system about food and body weight. In our culture, the valuing of thinness and the devaluing of fatness drive many people to unhealthy extremes in their relationship with food and body, such as repeated diets to achieve a weight goal that is unrealistic for them.

Other cultural factors that probably influence you are the prevalence of fast food restaurants, technology that minimizes the need for exercise, and customs centered on eating while socializing.

➤ How do you think cultural values and social customs affect your eating and weight?

➤ Write your ideas about *cultural/social* influences in **Petal C.**

● **D=Diet.** Think about your eating habits over the past two weeks. What is your typical pattern in terms of how, when, and what you eat? Do you snack all day long on potato chips and candy? Do you eat regularly, or skip meals often and then overeat at dinner?

If you analyzed your diet for a two week period and figured out the proportions of protein, complex carbohydrates, milk and dairy products, fresh fruits and vegetables, and fat that you ate, would it come close to the shape of the nutritional food pyramid, with the largest portion of foods eaten being carbohydrates, and the smallest being fat? Is your diet high in sugar, salt, fat, caffeine, or alcohol? How much water do you drink?

➤ How do you think your diet influences your food and weight problem?

➤ Write one or two examples of how your *diet* affects your food and weight problem in **Petal D.**

● **E=Emotional responses to food.** While eating in response to emotions is normal, it can become a problem if it's done too often. When you regularly eat in response to anger, loneliness, boredom, or stress, you are likely to gain weight, which can be frustrating (suddenly your clothes don't fit) and discouraging (you have worked so hard to maintain a healthy, stable weight). Taken to extremes, you might develop an eating disorder or mental health problem.

➤ How do your emotional responses to food affect your eating and body weight?

➤ Write examples of your *emotional responses to food* in **Petal E.**

● **F/G=Family history/genetics.** There is a strong genetic component to obesity, especially between mothers and daughters. If you are female and your mother and grandmother are large women, the chances are greater that you will also be large. All relatives contribute to your genetic history, so take a look at your family tree.

Besides body type, you may have inherited certain behaviors and attitudes about food, eating, and your body. Did anyone in your family have a weight problem, an eating disorder, or struggle with food? Did anyone in your family focus negatively on your eating, weight, or body size? What were your family rules or traditions about eating (eg, *Eat, drink, and be merry!* or *Overindulgence is sinful!*)?

➤ How do you think your family history has influenced your food or weight problems?

➤ Write examples of how you think *family history and genetics* influenced your food and weight problems in **Petal F/G.**

● **H=Hunger physiology.** Hunger and satiation are natural physiological states. When your body needs refueling, it gives hunger signals to alert you: an empty sensation or a rumbling, growling sound in your stomach that goes away when you eat. When the need is satiated, your brain signals back that your body has had enough, giving you a sensation of fullness.

In spite of biological messages from your body, signals of hunger and satiety are easy to miss, ignore, override, or confuse with other needs such as *psychological* hunger. When you have the urge to eat but are not truly hungry, it is usually *psychological* hunger, or a need to eat to reduce anxiety. In the extreme case of anorexia or chronic self-starvation, the person learns to ignore hunger sensations until the body actually shuts down.

  ➤ How do you think your *hunger physiology* influences your food and weight problems?

  ➤ Write examples of how you think your *hunger physiology* affects your food and weight problems in **Petal H.**

● **I=Intervening variables.** Many other life events can affect your eating and weight. Illness, injury, or medical treatments can cause you to gain or lose weight. Age, economics, work schedule, travel, geographic location, menopause, pregnancy, and other stressors can have a big impact.

  ➤ What other life events or changes do you think influence your food and weight problems?

  ➤ Write examples of other *intervening variables* that effect your food and weight problem in **Petal I.**

6. Ask participants if anyone still thinks problems with food and weight are simple. Invite comments and insights. Encourage participants to ask questions or share responses to their personal **Influencing Factors** picture.

7. Ask participants to reflect on the degree of influence each factor has on their food and weight problem.

  ➤ Look over the petals on your worksheet and think about the amount of influence each factor, **A** to **I,** has on you.

  ➤ Rank the factors in order of their influence on you, with #1 having the most influence and #8 having the least influence.

    ➤ Write your influencing factor hierarchy in the numbered spaces on your worksheet.

8. Invite participants to share examples of their most and least powerful influencing factors. Challenge the group to consider the relevance of their rankings to their decisions about what they will change.

  ● **Your most powerful influencing factors may or may not be the place to start.** On the other hand, these influences may hold the most energy or motivation for you to change. It's up to you to decide what you most want to change, and when.

9. Hand out additional copies of the **Influencing Factors** worksheet and invite participants to use them for taking notes while they explore possibilities for changing each factor.

☞ *Hang two sheets of newsprint for recording purposes. Divide each newsprint into four sections, so you have eight boxes, one for each of the eight categories of influencing factors. Label each box with the alphabetical letter that corresponds to that category.*

10. Invite participants to brainstorm ideas of possible strategies for changing each influencing factor. List ideas in the appropriate category box.

☞ *Come prepared with a list of ideas for each category: (A, walk to work instead of driving; B, eat less fat and exercise more often to reduce fat deposits; C, develop social activities that do not involve food, like playing a sport with friends, etc).*

11. Invite participants to look over all the strategies listed and select the ones that have the most potential to help them.

➤ Write a list of the most helpful strategies in the numbered spaces on your worksheet.

➤ Look over your list and circle one strategy that you would like to try this week.

12. Solicit examples of the kinds of strategies participants decided to try, and then encourage them to seek support in their efforts to change.

● **Support is a positive influencing factor for change.** Enlist support from family members, close friends, or other trusted people as you work on change. These connections will bolster and sustain you as you move from problems to solutions.

FOR ONGOING GROUPS

▓ Follow up this exercise at the next session by using **Influencing Factors** worksheets to focus on food and body issues in more depth. Each person puts her problem in the center and then explores all the factors that influence that issue in her life.

This exercise was contributed by Roxanne Bijold, RD.

INFLUENCING FACTORS

B
Body type

A Activity level

C Cultural/Social

I Intervening variables

FOOD and WEIGHT

PROBLEMS

D Diet

H Hunger
physiology

F/G
Family history /
Genetics

E Emotional
responses to food

1 _____

2 _____

3 _____

4 _____

5 _____

6 _____

7 _____

8 _____

10 CLEAN PLATE CLUB

The emotional issues of eating are put on the platter in this intriguing exploration of reasons for eating or not eating everything on your plate.

GOALS

To identify childhood messages about food and emotional issues that affect eating.

To develop strategies for changing patterns of overeating.

GROUP SIZE

Unlimited.

TIME FRAME

30–45 minutes.

MATERIALS NEEDED

Blank paper and **Clean Plate Club** worksheets; 2 newsprint sheets and 1 marker for each small group; masking tape.

PROCESS

1. Conduct an informal survey to determine how many group members are familiar with this topic.

   ✔ How many of you grew up in families that had a clean plate club?

   ✔ How many of you think you still belong to a clean plate club?

2. If appropriate, share a personal example of your own membership in this club. Then explain the nature of clean plate clubs in a chalktalk.

   ● **Clean plate clubs reflect the values of its members.** They are informal groups or systems (like families) which promote, praise, and reward you for eating everything on your plate. These groups associate clean plates with:

     ○ **Virtue** (you didn't waste a thing).
     ○ **Healthy nutrition** (you ate all your vegetables).
     ○ **Loyalty** (you never miss a Sunday dinner with your parents).
     ○ **Love** (you give and receive nurturance in the form of food).
     ○ **Affirmation** (it made the cook feel good when you asked for seconds and ate every last drop).

● While belonging to these clubs may bring pleasure, pride, and satis-faction, **membership may also bring physical and emotional pain.** Imagine the physical discomfort that you feel when you are utterly full and yet you continue to eat until you are stuffed. The long-term effects of doing this may result in an unwanted weight gain which may affect your health or self-esteem.

● **Club dues may include alienation from your body.** If it becomes a habit to tune out, ignore, or override the signals of your body when you have had enough, you may lose a vital connection to yourself and a trust in your body, at least in regard to its hungers.

● **Saying no to others is not easy.** Because food is such an important part of our cultural way of giving and receiving love, it can be very difficult for some people to leave food on their plates. Rejection of food, even when you've had enough, can be associated with rejection of friends, family, or even restaurant cooks and food servers who have worked hard to please you. Responses of others may range from friendly cajoling to eat more, to punitive shaming if you don't leave your plate shining clean.

● **Saying no to yourself can be just as hard.** Many people feel deprived if they don't eat everything available to them. This can be experienced as a rejection of yourself, since you are withholding something good from yourself. In this case, you keep yourself in the clean plate club to maintain status as a worthy, lovable person.

3. Divide the group into teams of four, asking participants to find three other people who typically eat off the same kind of plate (eg, pottery, plastic, paper, microwave trays, metal, china, etc). When everyone has found three companions, ask them to be seated in groups and give instructions for discussion.

➤ Take 2 minutes each to introduce yourself to your group and share your answers to these questions.

➢ Were you allowed to leave food on your plate as a child? Do you remember wanting to?

➢ What happened if you did or did not eat everything on your plate?

➤ Appoint a timekeeper.

4. After about 8 minutes, interrupt the group and invite participants to share examples of childhood consequences of not cleaning their plates. Relate these ideas to points made earlier in the chalktalk, especially those that illustrate the cultural and social pressures on people to eat everything on their plates.

☞ *Keep this discussion brief so the group energy does not diminish.*

5. Give each group two sheets of newsprint and a marker, then lead the groups in further exploration on this topic.

   ➤ Appoint the person who remembers licking their plate clean as a child to be group reporter.

   ➤ Brainstorm a list of messages you received as a child about food and eating.

      ➢ Include all ideas, both positive and negative.

      ➢ Reporters should write childhood messages down on one of the newsprints.

         ☞ *You may need to give examples: remember all the starving people in third world countries?*

   ➤ You have 5 minutes to make your list.

6. When 5 minutes are up, stop the discussions, and invite group reporters to come to the front of the room one at a time to share their group lists. Hang each newsprint with masking tape and when all group lists are posted, invite participants to reflect on the messages that are dominant for the whole group.

   ➤ Look over all the lists and find messages that are repeated more than once.

   ➤ Select the five most common messages and write them down on blank paper. These are the ones that hold the most power for this group.

   ➤ Now look over the list again, and pick the three that have the most influence on you *personally*.

      ➢ Write these down on your list of childhood messages about eating.

      ➢ If you think of other messages that have not been mentioned but which also affect your eating choices, add these to your list.

7. Distribute **Clean Plate Club** worksheets to each participant, and guide them through a step-by-step process for further reflection about the influence of different social situations on their eating patterns.

   ➤ Look over your worksheet and notice four empty plates. Imagine that you are going to have four separate meals in four different circumstances: at your parents' home, a friend's home, a restaurant, and with your current family, or, if you live alone, by yourself at home.

➤ Start with the first plate in the upper left corner. This is your parents' home. Imagine yourself eating a meal **with your parents.** (If your parents are deceased, imagine a meal shared when they were still alive, perhaps during childhood or early adulthood.)

➣ How much food will you leave on your plate? Think about your typical pattern, and draw in the portion that you will leave on your plate. If you will clean your plate, leave it blank.

➤ Now tune into the **feelings** you have about your eating choices. Do you feel satisfied? Angry? Guilty? Content? Uncomfortable?

➣ Write these feelings in the space below the plate.

➤ Focus on the **thoughts** you have about eating in this situation. What are you telling yourself about what you should or should not eat, and why? Refer to your list of childhood messages if you feel stuck.

➣ Write your thoughts in the space provided below the plate.

8. When participants have finished recording their reflections about the first meal, guide them through the remaining three meal scenarios, pausing after each step to allow time for group members to complete their worksheets.

➤ Move your attention to the second plate on the top right of your worksheet, which represents a meal **at your friend's house.**

➣ Take a minute to close your eyes and imagine this situation in your mind.

➣ Think about who you are with, what the surroundings are like, and any other details which will help you conjure up the mood and atmosphere of this setting.

➣ Decide how much food you will leave on your plate, using your typical responses in this situation as a guide for deciding.

➣ Draw in any leftover food on your plate.

➣ Record your feelings and thoughts about these choices in the spaces provided.

➤ Now move to the plate in the lower left corner of the worksheet, and imagine yourself eating a meal **in a restaurant.**

➣ Reflect on your typical pattern of eating in this situation, and draw in the amount of food you would leave on your plate, if any.

➣ Record your feelings and thoughts about the choices you made.

➤ Complete the fourth meal scenario on the bottom right of your worksheet, which is a meal with **your family at home** or, if you are single, a meal **by yourself at home.**

➤ Draw in the amount of food you would leave, if any, and record your feelings and thoughts in this circumstance.

9. When all have finished their worksheets, encourage participants to reflect further on their patterns, and to share their discoveries with members of their small group.

➤ Look over your worksheet and compare your eating patterns in these situations.

➤ Write down your observations and insights at the bottom of your worksheet.

➤ Share whatever you want about your four meal scenarios and how you did or did not participate in the clean plate club.

➤ Each person has 2 minutes to talk about your experiences.

➤ Other group members should listen attentively to each person, and refrain from giving advice or making judgements.

10. When everyone has had the opportunity to talk about their experiences, interrupt the discussions and invite participants to share with the larger group examples of common feelings and thoughts. Use these insights as a bridge to a short chalktalk pointing out the relationship between feelings, thoughts, and behavior.

● **Feelings and thoughts may determine our behavior—or be a consequence of actions already taken.** If you feel anxious and think that food will serve as a tranquilizer, you might decide to eat. This behavior may in turn trigger feelings of guilt or shame and thoughts about yourself as impulsive or weak.

● **The circular connection between feelings, thoughts, and behavior can be positive or negative.** When we speak of vicious circles, we are usually talking about a negative pattern such as fasting, overeating when under stress, and then regretting it afterwards. A positive cycle would be feeling hungry, eating food to satisfy this need, and recognizing how well you take care of yourself.

● **Ideally, we would eat when we were hungry and stop when we were full.** You would listen to your body and allow your physical need for nourishment, not emotional state or social setting, to guide your decisions about what, when, where, why, and how you eat.

11. Point out that everyone in the room has wisdom about how to stop overeating—and *resign* from the clean plate club. Challenge participants to work in their small groups to develop strategies that will help them curb overeating.

> Brainstorm a list of strategies for eating when you are hungry and stopping when you have had enough.

>> Identify ways to stop eating when you are *satisfied*, but not stuffed.

> Group reporters should record all ideas on the second sheet of newsprint.

> You have 5 minutes to develop your list.

12. When 5 minutes are up, ask group reporters to present their lists to the large group, and hang up each newsprint with masking tape. Summarize and affirm the creative ideas developed by participants, weaving them into a chalktalk offering tips for healthy, balanced eating.

● **Decide to respect and care for your body.** Be loyal to it. Listen to it. Feed it when it's hungry, but don't stuff it with food it doesn't want or need.

● **Relax before and during mealtimes.** Breathe deeply, release tension and stress, and slow down. Concentrate on the pleasure of eating without rush or distraction.

● **Practice leaving some food on your plate** when you have had enough. Experiment doing this in a variety of situations, and observe your own reactions as well as the reactions of other people. Record your reflections and observations regularly in a *food for thought journal*.

● **Practice taking smaller portions and eating slowly,** enjoying each bite. Wait before taking a second helping. Use a smaller plate to change your perception of portion size.

● **Learn to ignore or laugh off pressure from other people** to clean your plate. Practice simple responses, such as *Thanks, I'm satisfied*.

● **Address your own concerns about not cleaning your plate.** If you feel guilty about wasting food, save the leftovers for another time. If you worry about offending family or friends, reassure them of your enjoyment of their company while you assert your decision to say no to eating more food.

13. Invite participants to develop a plan for *resigning* from the clean plate club.

   ➤ Look over the strategy list again and pick out one or two strategies for overeating that you would like to try in the next month.

   ➤ Write a quick plan of action on the back of your worksheet.

14. Advise participants to follow their plans for at least one month. Then evaluate how well it's working.

FOR ONGOING GROUPS

   ■ Give additional blank worksheets to use as homework between sessions. Instruct participants to try out the four different meal scenarios and record their actions and reactions.

   ■ As a part of future meetings, include a routine discussion of how different strategies are working or not working.

   ■ Start a recipe file of winning strategies, and give 3x5 cards summarizing ideas to each participant.

© 1996 WHOLE PERSON PRESS 210 WEST MICHIGAN DULUTH MN 55802 ■ (800) 247-6789

CLEAN PLATE CLUB

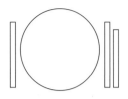

Parental Home

Feelings: _____

_____

_____

_____

Thoughts: _____

_____

_____

_____

_____

_____

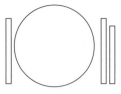

Home of Friend

Feelings: _____

_____

_____

_____

Thoughts: _____

_____

_____

_____

_____

_____

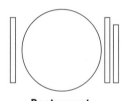

Restaurant

Feelings: _____

_____

_____

_____

Thoughts: _____

_____

_____

_____

_____

_____

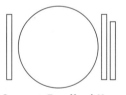

Current Family / Home

Feelings: _____

_____

_____

_____

Thoughts: _____

_____

_____

_____

_____

11 SENSATIONAL DIET

In this captivating exercise, participants go to a supermarket and shop for foods that will satisfy both physiological and psychological needs.

GOALS

To heighten awareness of the role of food texture in satisfying hunger.
To discover food choices that can satisfy cravings and nutritional needs.
To practice finding and comparing nutritional information about foods.

GROUP SIZE

Unlimited.

TIME FRAME

60–90 minutes.

MATERIALS NEEDED

Sensational Food List worksheets; newsprint; marker; masking tape or easel. Optional: $5.00 spending money for each of the four small groups. This can be provided by the leader or you could ask each participant to chip in $1.00 for their team purse.

PROCESS

☞ *This exercise requires a supermarket within walking distance or some arrangements for transportation. The process is designed for adaptation to nutritional information of the trainer's choice (eg, food exchanges, fat content, calorie content, etc). Customize the chalktalks, instructions, and worksheets to meet your educational objectives.*

1. Introduce the exercise with a brief chalktalk about the sensual nature of eating.

   ● **Eating is a sensual experience.** When we eat with full awareness, all our senses are involved. We are more likely to tune in to our hungers and satisfy them appropriately.

     ○ **Taste.** Foods are sweet, sour, spicy, salty, bitter, or some combination of these tastes. The tastes you enjoy will vary from day to day or month to month, depending on variables such as mood, physical health, age, life stress, sense of adventure, exposure, expanding palette, and many other factors.

○ **Smell.** The smell of food can start the saliva flowing and get the digestive juices moving in anticipation of what is to come. Or it can turn you away with a grimace.

○ **Touch.** How food feels in your mouth affects your enjoyment of it and your satisfaction after eating it. If you yearn for something chewy, pudding or broth just won't do it. If you want something crunchy and eat mashed potatoes, you'll be looking for more food after your meal is over, even if you're physically full.

○ **Sound.** Some foods are noisy, like chips and raw carrots. Remember the popularity of Rice Krispies with its *Snap, Crackle,* and *Pop* characters? It can be very satisfying to make a lot of noise when eating and to hear yourself munching away.

○ **Sight.** As with smell, the sight of food can trigger hunger responses, especially for people who are extra sensitive to visual food cues. Most people enjoy eating food that is attractively prepared and presented in an appealing manner.

● **Texture is an especially important variable for satisfying hunger.** Most people describe food by its texture, rather than its color or flavor. Common textures are *wet and crunchy* (eg, cucumbers, apples), *dry and crunchy* (eg, granola, taco chips), *chewy* (beef jerky, garlic bread), *soft and lumpy* (pasta, potato salad), and *creamy* (chocolate mousse, peanut butter).

Both physiological and emotional factors will pull you toward certain food textures on any given day. If you listen to your body and respond to these needs, you will find eating more pleasurable and satisfying.

2. Ask participants to reflect on the circumstances under which they are most likely to crave certain textures. Solicit a few examples.

✔ When are you most likely to crave *wet, crunchy food* like grapes? (eg, when hot and thirsty)

✔ When are you most likely to crave a *dry, crunchy food* like pretzels? (eg, when angry, tense, frustrated, or nervous)

✔ When are you most likely to crave a *chewy food* like caramels or bread? (eg, when emotions are running high or when needing a tension release)

✔ When are you most likely to crave a *soft, lumpy food* like baked beans or stewed tomatoes? (eg, when lonely or stressed out)

✔ When are you most likely to crave a *creamy food* like ice cream or yogurt? (eg, when needing comfort or nurturance)

3. Summarize the barriers against and the benefits of satisfying our sensual needs for certain foods.

● **Satisfying food texture needs is a challenge.** If you are stuck in an eating rut or are unaware of other available choices, you may unintentionally be depriving yourself of appealing textures. If you are trying to change your diet or eating habits for medical or health considerations, food choices—and textures—may be limited. If you are experimenting with giving yourself more freedom about eating, the abundance of choices may be overwhelming or scary.

● **Expanding sensory choices can lead to greater variety,** (which is healthy), an increased feeling of control (which makes you feel good), and a reduced risk of overeating or bingeing on the foods you crave (which is probably a habit you want to stop).

4. Announce that participants will go on a shopping trip to the local supermarket to scout out food choices in the five texture categories and then evaluate these options on the basis of nutritional value.

☞ *Insert a chalktalk on appropriate nutritional information here, adapting it to your chosen criteria (eg, RDA, average calories/serving, grams of fat/serving, sodium, vitamins, etc).*

5. Divide participants into five teams according to each type of food texture: wet and crunchy; dry and crunchy; chewy; soft and lumpy; and creamy. Give each team member their own **Sensational Food List** worksheet and explain the challenge for each team.

☞ *Instruct participants to label the columns to the right of the worksheet with nutritional values you have chosen for research (eg, fat grams, calories, sodium, etc).*

➤ Mark your group's texture category on the top of the worksheet.

➤ As a team, go to the supermarket and find as many foods as you can that will satisfy your **designated food texture criteria.**

➤ Visit every section of the store—from produce to canned goods to dairy to deli.

➤ Write every food you find on your **Sensational Food List** and record the nutritional values for each food item in the appropriate box on your worksheet.

➤ Seek a wide variety of foods without judging their nutritional value. Simply record the facts about each food.

➤ Spend 20 minutes finding foods. When the time is up, gather as a team at a designated place in the store, review your lists, and decide on one food item that you will buy as a representative sample of your texture category to share with other participants.

> Buy the chosen food item and return here.

> Ask someone to volunteer as team leader. This person will organize the team for scouting strategies at the store, keep track of time, collect team members' food lists at the end of the shopping trip, pay for chosen sample foods, and report back to the large group on team discoveries.

6. As teams return from the store, invite them to discuss the nutritional pros and cons of various foods in their texture group. Provide additional reference tools as needed.

7. After 5–10 minutes of nutritional analysis, invite team leaders to share insights, surprises, or discoveries about nutrition and their texture group.

8. Lead the participants in a personal reflection about their own food choices, habits, and considerations.

   > Which of the foods mentioned by each team do you already eat to satisfy these textual hungers?

   > Which foods would you choose not to eat because they are bad for your health?

   > Which foods offer new possibilities for satisfying both hunger and health considerations?

   ☞ *Point out that participants can refine their sensory selections by deciding whether they want the food hot or cold—or a combination of both.*

9. Invite participants to share examples of foods which they think may be helpful in satisfying complex hunger sensations, taking into account health considerations. Also solicit ideas from participants about food combinations that they have used successfully in the past for satisfying these needs.

10. Conclude with a chalktalk encouraging participants to continue building a **sensational diet.**

   ● **Make your diet as sensational as possible.** Food is intended to be satisfying. When you pay attention to your sensory experiences, you will become more and more skilled in giving yourself the physical and emotional nourishment you need.

FOR ONGOING GROUPS

■ Work on compiling a list of healthy, delicious substitutes for foods which participants crave but want to limit for medical or health reasons. Have participants try out the *substitute* foods one time and the *forbidden* foods another time. Encourage them to keep a journal of their level of satisfaction with each.

*Contributed by Julie Kembel, author of **Winning the Weight and Wellness Game** (Tuscon AZ: Northwest Learning Associates, 1993).*

SENSATIONAL FOOD LIST

Food Category   ___ wet and crunchy   ___ dry and crunchy   ___ chewy
___ soft and lumpy   ___ creamy

Food Item	Serving Size			

12 FOOD HOUSE FANTASY

This intriguing fantasy, based on the work of Carol H. Munter and Jane R. Hirschmann, will help participants discover what happens when they surround themselves with food they love.

GOALS

To discover how legalizing food affects appetite and cravings.
To reduce fears of food and hunger, and to relax around food.

GROUP SIZE

Unlimited.

TIME FRAME

45–60 minutes.

MATERIALS NEEDED

Blank paper; **Legalizing Food and Eating** worksheets; **Food House Fantasy** script; newsprint; markers.

PROCESS

☞ *This process is not appropriate for treatment or support groups based on an abstinence philosophy unless you are interested in helping participants explore the possibility of self-regulation.*

1. Distribute blank paper to everyone and give instructions for individual brainstorming.

   ➤ Think of all of the foods you *love* to eat.

      ➤ Temporarily set aside all of the judgments you usually have about food. Don't label any food as good/bad, healthy/unhealthy, nonfattening/fattening, legal/illegal, safe/dangerous.

      ➤ Make a list of all the foods that you enjoy—from ice cream to carrots to buttered popcorn to strawberries to sirloin steak.

2. After 3–4 minutes, solicit observations from the group on their internal censors.

   ✔ What judgements crept in as you made your list?

3. Reinforce the power these judgments have on our food choices, then guide participants in further reflection about their attitudes toward these favorite foods.

➤ Look back over your list.

➤ Put a *star* beside favorite foods you have in your home and allow yourself to enjoy regularly.

➤ Put a *circle* around favorite foods that you keep at arm's length, to be enjoyed only occasionally.

➤ *Underline* any favorite food that you will not allow yourself to eat under any circumstance.

4. Invite participants to share examples of foods they do not allow themselves to eat. These are foods we consciously or unconsciously label as dangerous, unhealthy, forbidden, illegal, fattening, or bad.

☞ *List all forbidden or restricted foods on newsprint.*

5. Conduct a survey about participants' attitudes and habits in regard to these restricted and/or forbidden foods.

✔ How many of you can find at least three foods in this restricted/ forbidden list that you absolutely love?

✔ How many of you avoid eating such foods that you love—or avoid having them in your home or workplace?

✔ How many of you feel anxious, guilty, or ashamed when you eat such foods?

✔ How many of you feel anxious, sad, or deprived when you *don't* eat these foods?

✔ How many of you crave these foods and/or binge on them?

6. Weave group responses into a chalktalk about legalizing food as an antidote for eating problems.

● One of the best **solutions for eating problems** of all types is to return all foods to a neutral status—to stop labeling foods as un- healthy/ healthy, bad/good, fattening/nonfattening, and to give yourself permission to eat all foods, trusting yourself to find a healthy balance. This process is called *legalizing foods.*

● **Legalizing food is more helpful than labeling.** Food categorizing usually backfires. The intent of labeling foods is to help people lose weight, but the polarizing of foods as either fattening or nonfat- tening turns millions of us into food junkies. Prohibition increases desire; nothing makes food more alluring than calling it forbidden.

● **Legalizing food is a means to an end.** The goal is to cure your eating problems, end your obsession with food and weight, and be at peace with food. You cannot do that as long as you evaluate food as either good or bad in terms of fat and calorie content.

● **Legalizing eating options is the opposite of dieting.** When you diet, you label certain food as fattening or forbidden—and then either restrict or deprive yourself of these foods. When you legalize food, you say *no* to diets forever. You make all foods equal in your mind, give yourself permission to eat when you are hungry, choose the food you are hungry for, and eat whatever quantity satisfies you. This process is called *demand feeding*. It involves learning to recognize internal hunger, eating whenever you feel hungry, and stopping when you've had enough.

● **Legalizing food requires action.** There are several things you will need to do:

○ Legalize food you love. Bring formerly forbidden foods into your home; surround yourself with foods you crave.

○ Replenish supplies of favorite foods. You should always keep an excess of what you need, so you'll never feel deprived.

○ Create a pleasant food atmosphere in your home. This means promising to stop yelling at yourself when you eat the food you love. Your goal is to legalize foods *and* eating.

7. Invite participants to share their concerns about legalizing food by asking them to complete this sentence: *If I legalize food, I'm afraid I will*. . . . List fears on newsprint, responding as appropriate with brief chalktalks.

● **Fear of losing control.** It is normal to be frightened of losing control and gorging on all the food you have brought into your house. Most people discover that when they surround themselves with great quantities of the foods they love and stop yelling at themselves for eating it, their craving diminishes almost immediately.

● **Gaining weight.** If you have just come off a diet, you may gain weight as part of a natural rebound from the dieting. Once you've truly legalized food, your weight should stabilize.

● **Wasting food.** The surplus of food is very important. It symbolizes caretaking, support, and permission to eat.

● **Health and nutrition.** If you have a medical condition (like diabetes) that responds to diet restrictions, you may need to modify your eating as a respectful response to your body's internal needs. Listening to your body is very different from imposing external judgements that declare certain foods bad or forbidden.

● **Protecting your food supply.** You need to know that your food will be there when you want it. If other family members eat it, your caretaking process is sabotaged. Find a special cupboard or shelf for *your* food and explain to family members the reasons they cannot eat it. Each family member can have his or her own shelf if you want.

8. Announce that participants will have the opportunity to fantasize about what might happen if they legalize food in their life. Encourage everyone to find a comfortable position or place in the room and, when everyone is settled in, read the **Food House Fantasy** script.

9. Invite participants to share examples of what happened in their fantasy experience. Help volunteers clarify the implications of their fantasy, in terms of what they need to do to legalize foods they crave, replenish supplies of foods they love, and create a pleasant food atmosphere in their home.

10. Hand out **Legalizing Food and Eating** worksheets and encourage participants to think about what they need to do to legalize food and eating.

    ➤ Think about the foods you love and your experience in the **Food House Fantasy.**

    　➤ Do you have these foods in your home?

    　➤ Is your supply of these foods restricted or running out?

    　➤ What foods do you need to restore to your cupboards?

    　➤ Record these on the top of your worksheet as foods you will buy.

    ➤ Think of the changes you need to make to create a more pleasant food environment in your home.

    　➤ Do you need to organize your kitchen, decorate your dining room, make your meals more appealing?

    　➤ Write or draw your ideas in the middle of your worksheet.

    　　☞ *Allow 4–5 minutes for participants to complete their worksheets.*

    ➤ At the bottom of the page, write a phrase or motto which will give you permission and encouragement to eat the food you love. For example, *Hearty appetite! Enjoy, enjoy; Feed yourself with care; Savor and satisfy;* or *Trust myself!* are phrases which express support for eating and enjoying food.

11. Invite participants to share their plans with another person.

    ➤ Pair up with another person you do not know well.

    　➤ Decide who will be *Fantasy* and who will be *Reality.*

➤ **Fantasy** goes first. Describe your food house fantasy and your plans for legalizing food and eating while **Reality** listens and supports your ideas.

➤ After 3 minutes, reverse roles. **Reality** share your food house fantasy and legalizing plans while **Fantasy** listens.

☞ *Announce when 3 minutes are up and it's time to switch roles.*

12. Invite participants to share their plans and mottos for legalizing food and eating.

13. Conclude with a chalktalk outlining cautions about legalizing food.

   ● **Legalizing food is not an end in itself.** Remember that this process is a means to an end: freedom from eating problems; an end to obsessions with food, weight, and body image; and unconditional self-care.

   ● **Attend to issues other than food.** When you legalize food and take away its power to make you feel bad, you will be left with the same issues or bad feelings about yourself that started you dieting in the first place. Without the distraction of food/body obsessions, these issues and feelings may surge up with new intensity. Attend to them, surround yourself with support, seek professional help if you need it.

14. For more information on this topic, refer participants to *Overcoming Overeating* and *When Women Stop Hating Their Bodies* by Jane R. Hirshmann and Carol H. Munter.

FOR ONGOING GROUPS

▓ Plan a group food feast. Have participants bring in their favorite foods, eat a meal together, and then process their feelings about the experience. Those who are not hungry can wrap up food to eat later.

▓ Have participants enact their plan to legalize food and eating as homework. If legalizing all foods is too scary, have them try just one food to start. Talk about how it went at the next session.

▓ Have participants bring in one formerly forbidden food and use it to create an art form that symbolizes their freedom from fear of this food.

This exercise was contributed by Jane R. Hirschmann and Carol H. Munter, authors of **Overcoming Overeating** *and* **When Women Stop Hating Their Bodies,** *who orginated the concept of legalizing food.*

© 1996 WHOLE PERSON PRESS 210 WEST MICHIGAN DULUTH MN 55802 ■ (800) 247-6789

FOOD HOUSE FANTASY

Make yourself as comfortable as possible . . .
Settle back . . . close your eyes . . . and take a deep breath . . .
Slowly exhale . . .
and allow yourself to focus on the regular, easy rhythm of your breathing.
Continue to relax . . . and enjoy the quiet, calm sound of your breathing . . .
allowing yourself to let go of tension . . .
as you slow yourself down . . . and focus on this moment.
Imagine yourself alone in a beautiful meadow filled with wildflowers . . .
and the sound of birds singing . . .
The sun warms your skin . . .
and you are struck by the beauty of all that surrounds you.

☞ *Pause 10 seconds.*

You see a path leading from the meadow into a wooded area . . .
and you decide to follow it . . .
The woods are damp, plush, and green . . . filled with the rich aroma of pine.
The path narrows, but you continue to follow it.
Up ahead, in a clearing lit by streaks of sunlight . . . you see a house.
As you approach, you notice a sign over the front door.
On the sign is your name and the words Food House.

☞ *Pause 10 seconds.*

Open the front door and walk in.
Inside you find a house filled with all the foods you have ever wanted . . .
Savor the sight of all your favorite foods gathered here . . . just for you.

☞ *Pause 5 seconds.*

As you explore the house . . . allow the accumulated tension of years of
denial and self-control to drain away . . .
as you realize that you have found a treasure . . .
Look around . . . take your time . . . you have as long as you need.

☞ *Pause 20 seconds.*

When you decide to leave, remember that you can return whenever you want.
You know what this house is. You know how to find it.
Now, go to the meadow and rest a while.
Then, when you are ready, open your eyes.

This fantasy was contributed by Jane R. Hirschmann and Carol H. Munter, from their book **When Women Stop Hating Their Bodies** *(New York: Fawcett Columbine, 1995).*

LEGALIZING FOOD AND EATING

Foods I will buy for myself

Changes I will make to create a pleasant food environment

Motto

13 SPIRITUAL HUNGER

In this three-part exercise, participants identify spiritual hunger and thirst, imagine ways to satisfy hunger and thirst, and express gratitude for their fulfillment.

GOALS

To identify spiritual hunger and thirst.

To create imagery of a feast that satisfies the longing of the soul.

To celebrate with a simple ritual of thanksgiving.

GROUP SIZE

Unlimited.

TIME FRAME

60–90 minutes.

MATERIALS NEEDED

Copy of **Psalm 63** (p. 60) and a **Spiritual Hungers** worksheet for each participant; art materials (pastels, watercolors, magazines for collages, clay, etc); tissues; pitchers of ice water; fresh fruits; wholesome breads; table and cloth; CD or cassette player; taped meditative music (eg, *Pachelbel Canon in D;* Windham Hill *Winter Solstice*).

PROCESS

☞ *This exercise presumes the ability or agility to move from the desert experience to the oasis experience. This is essentially a leap of faith, one that follows an ancient pattern outlined in many of the psalms in the Hebrew Scriptures. You will use a psalm as a model for this movement. If individuals are not comfortable with the imagery of God as the One who satisfies their longing, you may suggest some alternative imagery.*

1. Invite participants to find a relaxed and comfortable position for a 5-minute meditative period. Distribute handouts of **Psalm 63**. Tell the group you will read through the first verse very slowly, three times. Then explain how they should continue the meditation once you have stopped reading.

   ➤ After the third reading aloud, read **Psalm 63, v. 1** silently to yourself, until the words of the first verse become like a breath prayer.

      ➤ Breathe slowly and deeply.

➤ Let the words of the psalm float over the top of your breathing. Start the music and read **Psalm 63, v. 1** three times. Read slowly and without much inflection.

☞ *This is a Benedictine practice for daily reading of the Scriptures. The calm and quiet intonation of the words give each individual a chance to apprehend the Holy in their own way.*

2. Allow 5 minutes for quiet. Then close the meditation time by reading **Psalm 63, v. 1** aloud one more time.

3. Introduce the reflection time with the observation that hunger and thirst are often signs of an unsatisfied spiritual need. Challenge participants to identify particular cravings or appetites that may be signs of a spiritual hunger. Hand out **Spiritual Hungers** worksheets and give suggestions on how to identify spiritual hungers.

   ➤ Write, paint, draw, sculpt, or make a collage that completes one or more of the sentences on the worksheet.

   ➤ Be creative and trust your intuition. Whatever medium you choose is fine.

   ☞ *As people get in touch with the depth of some of these needs, there may be tears. Prepare for this by promoting a safe space for reflection and providing tissues.*

   ➤ You have 15 minutes to work on your creative answers or images.

4. When 15 minutes are up, ask participants to talk about their spiritual hungers with another group member.

   ➤ Pair up with a neighbor and share your discoveries about your spiritual hunger.

   ➤ Each person has 3 minutes to talk about their creations.

5. Give a short chalktalk about the possibility of using this verse for coping with future struggles in their lives.

   ● **Commit this verse to memory.** It will be there for you to repeat silently to yourself when you find yourself in an emotional desert. It can also break the chain of compulsive eating or drinking as it stops you from reaching for something that does not really satisfy.

   ● **Identify the satisfaction** that can come from acknowledging God's presence or help, the fulfillment of a feast that results from celebrating with another, or singing a joyful tune, or being awakened to the beauty of Creation, or of a good wholesome meal that is eaten with appreciation and gratitude for the textures and tastes and holiness of table fellowship.

© 1996 WHOLE PERSON PRESS 210 WEST MICHIGAN DULUTH MN 55802 ■ (800) 247-6789

6. Invite participants to join in another 5-minute meditative exercise. Encourage everyone to get comfortable and, when people are settled, explain that this visualization will take place as you read the next segment of **Psalm 63**. Remind participants of the process.

   ➢ After I've read the passage aloud three times, read **Psalm 63, verses 5–6** silently to yourself.

   ➢ Breathe slowly and let the words become breath.

   Play the music and read **Psalm 63, verses 5–6** three times.

7. After a few minutes of silence, read through the verses one more time. Then ask people to envision the feast that satisfies them.

   ➢ Imagine the feast that satisfies you.

   ➢ Is it a table laden with your favorite foods?
   ➢ Is it a long sleep in a sun-dappled hammock?
   ➢ Is it a celebration with friends?
   ➢ A concert of sacred music?
   ➢ An answered prayer?
   ➢ A long hike outdoors?
   ➢ What satisfies your soul?

8. Invite participants to form small groups of 3–4 people to share their visualizations.

   ➢ Share as much as you are comfortable disclosing about your spiritual feast.

   ➢ Make a commitment to satisfy your hunger by pursuing your vision.

   ➢ Set a date or a time and tell others in your group how you will accomplish this.

9. After about 6–8 minutes, give a brief chalktalk about gratitude as a model of health that naturally follows desire and fulfillments.

   ● **Gratitude is the final step to fulfilling our hungers.** One of the models of health that comes in the Psalmist's movement from desire to fulfillment is the gratitude that is expressed—*the joyful praising with joyful lips*. Identify the longing, visualize what you need, realize (or make a commitment to realize) that fulfillment, and then give thanks.

10. Reconvene the group and indicate that you are going to have a feast of thanksgiving, a simple celebration with cold water, fresh fruit, and wholesome breads. Have participants sit in a circle and encourage them to serve one another.

➤ Share something for which your are grateful.

➤ Toast each other.

➤ Enjoy your thanksgiving feast.

11. Encourage participants to satisfy their spiritual hunger in the ways they have planned. Give a final, brief chalktalk to remind them that the final step of the exercise is that of praise and thanksgiving.

● **Thankfulness is the final course of this feast.** Expressions of gratitude are an important ending to the satisfaction of your hungers.

FOR ONGOING GROUPS

▨ This exercise is best suited for groups that have already established trust.

▨ Have participants start a *spiritual hunger journal,* noting spiritual yearnings or fulfillment and gratitude as they occur. Encourage daily meditation and journaling.

This exercise was contributed by Laura Loving.

PSALM 63*

Psalm 63, v. 1   *O God, you are my God,*
I seek you, my soul thirsts for you,
my flesh faints for you,
as in a dry and weary land
where there is no water.

vs. 5–6   *My soul is satisfied with a rich feast,*
and my mouth
praises you with joyful lips
when I think of you on my bed,
and meditate on you in the watches of the night.

*New Revised Standard Version.

SPIRITUAL HUNGERS

When I want comfort food I'm also hungry for . . .
(eg, something spiritual in nature such as reassurance, a sense of my place on the planet, God's presence, etc).

_____

_____

_____

When I experience emptiness, I am looking for . . .

_____

_____

_____

When I want to drown my sorrows, I need . . .

_____

_____

_____

When I want to reward myself, I'm seeking . . .

_____

_____

_____

When I need a jolt of caffeine, I could also use . . .

_____

_____

_____

14 FOOD: THE FEELING PLUG

People who use food as a way to cope with feelings discover alternatives for expressing emotions and nurturing themselves.

GOALS

To understand personal associations between moods and foods.

To develop natural alternatives to eating when feelings are strong.

To affirm the value of healthy expression of feelings.

GROUP SIZE

Unlimited.

TIME FRAME

30–40 minutes.

MATERIALS NEEDED

Foods and Moods worksheets; newsprint and marker.

PROCESS

1. Start by polling the group about *emotional eating* and asking for examples.

    ✔ How many of you think you eat, at least sometimes, in response to feelings other than hunger?

    ✔ What are your emotional eating patterns?

2. Weave responses into a chalktalk about emotional eating.

    ● **Most people eat to soothe their feelings, at least occasionally.** This response is common enough to be considered unavoidable and normal. A snack during times of stress may help you calm down— and provide renewed energy for coping with daily stress.

    ● **Eating in response to stress is often learned.** Early childhood experience may lead you to associate food with caretaking, comfort, and love. If your family was troubled, you may have turned to food for self-care or as a soothing tonic for pain. These are valid coping responses and should not be judged as bad since they helped you to survive in a difficult environment.

    ● **Emotional eating can cause problems.** While food may be a temporary balm for emotional upsets, it does carry risks for added complications in your life.

○ **Repression of healthy emotions.** Expressing our feelings in an appropriate and timely manner is essential for mental and physical health. Consider, for example, the benefits of talking through conflicts instead of repressing anger: reduced blood pressure, fewer physical symptoms of tension and pain in your body, increased intimacy in your relationships, and the overall sense of relief you feel when you have been honest, cleared the air, and let go of resentment. These benefits are lost if you bury your feelings in food.

○ **Ignoring other problems that need attention.** If we eat when we are bored or lonely, we may not address the problem of emptiness or loneliness in our lives. If you devour a bag of chips when you are furious with a friend, you may not resolve the conflict that caused your anger. If you hide your tears in a bowl of popcorn, you may postpone healing your grief or coming to peace with your losses.

○ **Developing a problematic relationship with food.** Emotional eating may lead to compulsive overeating, chronic dieting, binge-eating, bulimia, or anorexia. Your body may suffer from repeated dietary changes, malnutrition, or other health issues. These problems may range from mild upsets such as indigestion, to severe, life-threatening illnesses like anorexia.

○ **Relying on a single method of coping with stress.** We need multiple skills to manage stress: relaxation, problem solving, support, movement, expression of feelings, assertiveness, and many more. When food is your only resource—or eating is your favorite method of coping—you are painfully undernourished in your stress management menu. This would be like allowing yourself one kind of food, day after day. Just as you need a variety of nutritious foods every day, you need a mixture of coping skills to thrive.

3. Hand out **Foods and Moods** worksheets and guide participants through a reflection about their own connections between mood and food.

➤ In the first column, labeled **Moods,** star those you commonly experience (eg, today, this week). Feel free to add other typical moods for you.

☞ *For this and each succeeding reflection allow 1–2 minutes for participants to complete the worksheet step, then give the next instruction. Feel free to add any moods to the list.*

➤ Now go back and consider each mood you starred and the food you associate with that mood. In the second column, labeled **Foods,** write the first food that comes to your mind for each starred mood. For example, if your mood is *sad* and you think of chocolate cake, write this down. If your mood is *mad* and you think of a good stiff drink, record this association.

➤ In the third column, labeled **Activities** on your worksheet, list the first physical action that comes to your mind for each mood. For example, if your mood is *happy* you might dance or sing. If your mood is *mad,* you might yell or chop weeds in your garden.

4. Invite participants to consider what might happen if they severed the mood-food connection and created a mood-activity connection instead.

   ➤ Cross out the entire second column and graphically connect each starred mood with its corresponding action.

5. Conduct a survey to determine which moods are the most difficult for participants to handle.

6. Select the 3–5 most difficult moods and divide participants into small groups focused on these emotions, allowing participants to choose the group most relevant to them.

   ☞ *Allow groups as small as two or as large as eight people. If more than eight people want to work on the same emotion, form a second or third group.*

7. When everyone has joined a group, pass out newsprint and markers to each group and give instructions for introductions.

   ➤ Introduce yourself to the group by sharing the food-mood association you have for the emotion chosen by your group.

   ➤ The person with the sweetest food association is appointed timekeeper.

   ➤ Each person has 1 minute to explain why this emotion is especially hard for you to handle.

8. When most groups have finished introductions, interrupt with further instructions.

   ➤ Brainstorm a list of actions *other than eating* that you can do whenever you feel this mood.

   ➤ Think of realistic, practical things you can do easily on any given day. Be sure to share activities from your worksheet.

➤ You have 5 minutes to create your list.

➤ The person who experienced this emotion most recently is appointed group recorder.

➤ Recorders write all group ideas on newsprint and report back to the large group on results of the brainstorming.

9. When 5 minutes are up, invite group recorders up to the front of the room to share their group action strategies. Hang the lists and encourage participants to take notes on ideas generated by all groups.

☞ *Look for the strategy of **doing nothing** or **riding out the feelings**. If this is not mentioned by anyone be sure to point this out as a valid option in your summary chalktalk.*

10. Invite participants to identify any ideas which they think are not realistic. Discuss issues raised by the group and then encourage participants to reflect on strategies most helpful to them.

➤ Look over the list again and make note of the actions you think would be most helpful to you in handling this emotion.

11. Weave group responses into a closing chalktalk about how to care for your moods without turning to food.

● **Practice identifying your moods.** Give yourself attention. Stop what you are doing, do a mood check by asking yourself what you are feeling and then quickly brainstorm six possible actions for handling this mood. Make sure that you have at least five non-eating choices. *I could . . . or . . . or . . . or . . . or . . .*

● **Experiment with different actions for handling your moods.** Become a neutral observer of yourself. What happens when you are tired, do you walk instead of eat? What is it like to sit still, close your eyes, and relax when you are scared instead of seeking a comfort food?

● **Remember that doing nothing can also be a self-care action.** You can stop trying to block or control feelings. By doing nothing, you can simply notice your feelings and allow them to be. Let them run their course through your body. They may pass through you in waves, change in intensity, and then diminish or go away altogether.

● **Give yourself some slack.** We all eat in response to emotions sometime. When you do this, go easy on yourself. This is a time to remind yourself of your humanity and care for yourself unconditionally.

FOR ONGOING GROUPS

▣ Use the **Foods and Moods** worksheet as homework between session.

▣ Work on identification, expression, and validation of feelings in the group. Practice naming feelings and acting them out appropriately and constructively in group, through group process, role play, or psychodrama.

▣ Expand food-mood associations by adding thoughts about body size, dieting, bingeing, or other eating conflicts that are triggered by mood. For example, sadness might be associated with craving chocolate and body hatred.

This exercise was contributed by Lucia Capacchione.

FOODS AND MOODS

MOODS	FOODS	ACTIVITIES
lonely	_____	_____
grouchy	_____	_____
elated	_____	_____
nervous	_____	_____
sad	_____	_____
excited	_____	_____
discouraged	_____	_____
confident	_____	_____
bored	_____	_____
jealous	_____	_____
happy	_____	_____
irritable	_____	_____
anxious	_____	_____
hopeful	_____	_____
mad	_____	_____
angry	_____	_____
scared	_____	_____
confused	_____	_____
worried	_____	_____
disappointed	_____	_____
furious	_____	_____
relaxed	_____	_____
relieved	_____	_____
ashamed	_____	_____
frustrated	_____	_____
_____	_____	_____
_____	_____	_____
_____	_____	_____

15 WHOLE PERSON SNACK PACK

Compulsive overeaters, chronic dieters, and people seeking to break free of food obsessions will find the *whole person snack pack* an essential antidote, while normal eaters will find it practical, healthful, and satisfying.

GOALS

To explore strategies for stopping compulsive overeating and reestablishing normal eating patterns.

To reestablish a connection between food and physiological hunger.

To gain skill in self-nurturing.

GROUP SIZE

Unlimited.

TIME FRAME

45–60 minutes.

MATERIALS NEEDED

Whole Person Snack Pack worksheets; VHS VCR and monitor; *The Anti-Diet Diet* (10–minute segment from *The Losing Game,* a 50-minute video, available from Allbritton TV Productions, ATTN: Jane Cohen, 3007 Tilden St NW, Washington DC 2008, 1-202-364-7889; purchase cost $24.95); newsprint and marker.

PROCESS

☞ *This process assumes that the trainer is advocating a non-dieting approach by legalizing all foods and encouraging participants to eat what they want, when they want, until they are satisfied.*

1. Poll the group to get a sense of participants' attitudes about diets.

   ✔ How many of you have been on diets in the past?

   ✔ How many of you are convinced they don't work?

   ✔ How many of you are trying to legalize food and eat *normally—* only in response to physiological hunger?

2. Point out that the numbers of participants who want to stop dieting and return to eating spontaneously is reflective of a larger, nationwide movement against dieting. Announce that you have a 10-minute clip from a video called *The Losing Game* that you want to show

participants, and then start the video segment titled *The Anti-Diet Diet.*

3. Invite participants to share their reactions to the video, and then give a chalktalk summarizing the process of changing from a dieting pattern to a normal eating pattern, focusing on the principles of *natural eating* and *wholistic self-care.*

- **Stop dieting.** Throw away your scales, calorie counters, and other diet gadgets and gimmicks. Decide to never go hungry or deprive yourself of food again. Choose to embark on the adventure of feeding yourself on *all* levels: physically, mentally, spiritually, and socially.

- **Normalize food, eating, and self-care.** All foods are equal, regardless of calories or nutritional value. No food is off limits, bad, or forbidden. Food is just food. Once food is put in its natural place, it is no more or less important than other sources of nourishment. Play, laughter, work, intimacy, friendship, relaxation, creativity, exercise, and social support all contribute to your health and well-being.

- **Be generous with yourself.** Keep an ample, *accessible* supply of foods you love, and nonfood snacks that nourish and revitalize you. If you love hot soup, carry a small thermos with you to work. If you hunger for daily movement, plan time for stretching, walking, swimming, or other activities that you love. Replace self-neglect or deprivation with self-care, and strive for healthy balance in your life.

- **Tune in to your internal hunger.** Become a responsive listener to your biological hunger, and learn how to separate it from your psychological, spiritual, social, emotional, and mental hunger. Are you hungry for food in your stomach or your mind? Do you need something meaty like a hamburger, or do you need time to chew over a perplexing problem or challenge at work? The goal is to recognize the kind of hunger you have and, if possible, satisfy it.

- **Develop tolerance of yourself.** It takes time to develop consistent, appropriate self-care habits. If you snack on food when you are really hungry for a friendly talk with a friend, don't despair. It is normal to fall into old habits when you are trying to develop new patterns. Practice being sympathetic and patient with yourself.

- **Fine tune your skills.** The more you practice responding to your hungers, the more adept you'll become in figuring out exactly what you need, when you need it, and how much you need. You will become an excellent self-nurturer and a loving parent to yourself.

Over time, this will become more natural to you and will take less time and energy.

4. Invite questions about spontaneous eating and wholistic self-care, and then guide participants in a mini-exercise to recognize their hunger and its location in their body.

➤ Close your eyes, take a few deep breaths, and relax.

➤ Place your hand on your abdomen, just below your belly button, and tune in to your internal hunger.

➤ Decide how hungry you are on a scale of 0–10, with *0* being *famished* and *10* being *stuffed so full you can't move.*

➤ When you have rated your hunger level, focus on where the hunger sensation is located.

➤ Do you feel it in your stomach or your mouth?

➤ Do you have the urge to eat at this moment?

➤ If you are hungry, what food would satisfy you? Something hot, cold, wet, dry, crunchy or creamy, sweet or sour?

➤ If you are not hungry but feel the urge to eat, what do you want? What other things besides food would satisfy this craving?

5. Ask participants to share their experiences in identifying current hunger sensations, and clear up any confusion about the difference between stomach hunger and mouth or soul hunger. Then point out the benefits of responding appropriately to various hungers.

● **Basic self-care involves feeding yourself when you are hungry.** Ideally, this is within 10 minutes of receiving a strong hunger signal from your stomach. It also means feeding yourself the foods you are hungry for, regardless of their practicality or conformation to societal norms about what, when, or where to eat. It means eating a baked potato or sandwich for breakfast at the office if it suits your hunger cycle, or cereal and fruit for supper if this is what satisfies you.

● **Recognizing and responding to internal hunger builds security** and trust in yourself. When you listen to your hunger and make efforts to satisfy it, you send yourself (and others) the powerful message that you matter—that your needs are important—and that you can take care of yourself. It also builds confidence that you can trust yourself with food because regular, dependable feeding when you are hungry will stop the diet/binge cycle.

- **There are health benefits to eating more often.** Eating smaller meals more frequently aids in digestion, keeps blood sugar stable, reduces fatigue, enables your body to metabolize food more efficiently, and helps prevent overeating and weight gain. By paying attention to the daily rhythms of your hunger, you can learn to maximize energy throughout the day by refueling when your body needs it.

- **Eating in response to hunger takes planning.** Whenever your stomach starts grumbling, you need to be prepared with an appropriate snack. Having a food pack at work, in the car, and in your briefcase, allows you to refuel easily under any circumstances.

6. Hand out **Whole Person Snack Pack** worksheets and guide participants through a reflection about the kinds of food and nonfood items they could carry for daily nourishment.

   ➤ Assume that you are the most loving, attentive, sympathetic parent you could possibly be for yourself.

   ➤ Think about filling your food pack with both food and nonfood items that would nourish you on a given day.

      ➢ What foods are you likely to want? Will you want something hot like a cup of soup—or cold and creamy like yogurt? Will you need something thick and chewy like french bread—or thin and crunchy like crackers or pretzels? What about your sweet tooth? And what will satisfy your thirst?

      ➢ What nonfood items do you need? A book of affirmations or a prayer? A cassette player and tape with environmental sounds for a 10-minute relaxation break? Comfortable shoes for a noontime walk? The phone number of a friend? A good mystery novel? A journal to keep track of your stomach and mouth hunger experiences?

   ➤ Write or draw in all of the food and nonfood items you want in your **Whole Person Snack Pack.**

      ➢ Make every effort to incorporate all the things that will nourish you, even if doing so requires extra planning and preparation.

7. Ask participants to pair up with another participant to share the contents of their snack pack.

   ➤ Show your partner your snack pack, describe all of its contents, and explain why you chose to include these specific items.

   ➤ Each person has 2 minutes to share their snack pack contents.

---

8. Invite participants to share examples of the contents of their snack packs. Solicit a wide variety of examples of both food and nonfood items.

9. Ask participants to brainstorm a list of barriers to carrying a snack pack and list these obstacles on newsprint.

   ☞ *Be sure that the common barriers of embarrassment and resentment are included on the list.*

10. Give a brief chalktalk about two common barriers to carrying a snack pack: embarrassment and resentment.

    ● **Embarrassment has to do with entitlement.** If you believe you have the right to eat, you won't feel embarrassed about doing it in public. You don't lose the right to eat if your body is large, any more that you lose the right to breathe or sleep.

    ● **Resentment has to do with unmet childhood needs.** Feeding yourself may remind you of past hungers—physical and psychological—that went unnoticed or unsatisfied by your parents. It may make you angry that you have to parent yourself now, as an adult. It doesn't seem fair. But once you work through these feelings, you'll be able to experience the satisfaction and joy that comes from nurturing yourself.

11. Conclude by encouraging participants to carry a snack pack every day. This sends the powerful message that they can care for themselves and trust themselves to respond to their own needs—and that they are worthy of all this attention!

FOR ONGOING GROUPS

■ Encourage participants to bring their snack packs to group meetings and eat whenever they are hungry.

■ Have participants keep a log of their hunger levels, recording when they experience stomach hunger and when they feel mouth hunger, so they can understand the difference and practice eating only in response to stomach hunger.

WHOLE PERSON SNACK PACK

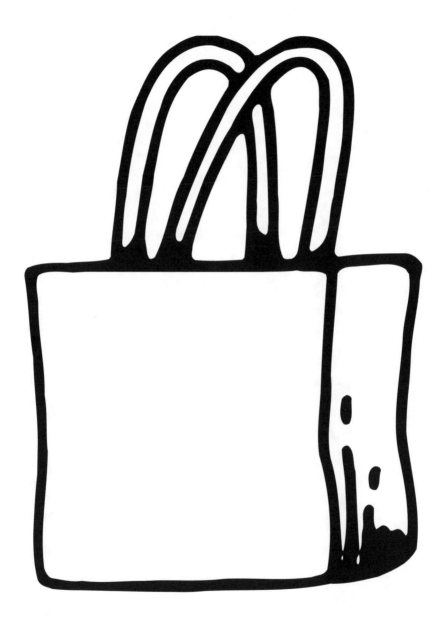

16 IDEAL PATTERNS

Participants examine normal and abnormal patterns of eating and exercising, then use an acronym to identify ideal patterns for sustenance, pleasure, and satisfaction.

GOALS

To recognize normal and abnormal patterns of eating and exercising.

To identify personal habits of eating and exercising that are healthy, unhealthy, or ideal.

GROUP SIZE

Unlimited.

TIME FRAME

45–60 minutes.

MATERIALS NEEDED

Newsprint and marker; blank sheets of paper.

PROCESS

1. Start with a chalktalk defining normal and abnormal.

   ● **Normal and abnormal are relative concepts,** dependent on the social and cultural standards or the environment. *Normal* means conforming to the standard of common type; whereas *abnormal* means not typical or usual, or deviating from a standard or norm. What is normal for one culture may be abnormal for another. For example, witchcraft was considered abnormal by European colonists in the 18th century, but it is normal for the Zulu people of South Africa in the 20th century.

   ● **Families teach about normal eating and exercising.** Parents teach us what is okay and not okay—from eating patterns to body attitudes. If you were forced to eat your vegetables *no matter what,* you were taught to abuse your body for the sake of nutrition or health. If you were given candy and cookies every time you felt hurt, you were taught to use food for comfort. If you grew up in a family of athletes, you were taught that exercise is natural. Most of us have a distorted picture of what is normal and abnormal, especially in relation to food, eating patterns, body image, and exercise. If you saw your mother dieting year after year, exercising as a punishment for eating, you learned to value thinness more than enjoyment of life.

2. Ask participants to brainstorm characteristics of normal eating and exercising patterns, write them on newsprint, and hang them on a blackboard or wall.

☞ *Make sure diverse qualities or characteristics of normal eating and exercise are included.*

Normal eating *behavior*
- *eating foods you like and enjoy*
- *no forbidden foods unless you have a medical condition that necessitates restriction*
- *ability to use moderate restraint to ensure nutritious diet, but not so restrictive that you miss out on pleasurable food*
- *three meals a day most of the time, but can also be several small meals throughout the day*
- *eating in response to internal hunger*
- *eating sometimes in response to mood or emotions*
- *sometimes eating it all because it tastes delicious*

Normal exercise *qualities*
- *based on enjoyable activity that energizes you*
- *does not cause you pain*
- *done in moderation (no more than 1 hour/day, 5 days/week on average)*
- *sometimes overdoing it and getting sore*
- *sometimes underdoing it and getting lethargic*
- *permission not to exercise when you are feeling ill, exhausted, or out of sorts*
- *movement that will increase heart rate but keep it in a healthy target zone (so you are slightly breathless but can still carry on a conversation)*
- *warming up and cooling down before and after exercise*

Normal eating *and* normal exercise
- *is a health issue, not a moral issue*
- *is flexible, not rigid*
- *is based on trust of body*
- *takes up some time and attention, but is not the only important thing in your life*
- *varies in response to emotions, energy, hunger, opportunity, and lifestyle*

3. Point out the themes of normal eating and exercise: it's done in moderation and is flexible, pleasurable, variable, and balanced with other parts of your life. Ask participants to think about whether these pat-terns were considered normal in their families.

4. Ask participants to brainstorm characteristics of abnormal eating and exercising, write these on newsprint, and hang them beside the list of normal eating and exercise patterns.

   ☞ *Make sure diverse characteristics of abnormal eating and exercise are mentioned.*

   ### Abnormal eating *behaviors*
   - *eating when not hungry*
   - *often eating in response to emotions (anger, sadness, loneliness, boredom)*
   - *continuing to eat after your body feels full*
   - *feeling out of touch with your body signals of fullness and hunger*
   - *eating or not eating to punish your body*
   - *rigidly counting calories, fat grams, etc, every time you eat*
   - *feeling guilty or anxious if you eat something fattening*
   - *making yourself throw up or use laxatives to make up for mistakes in eating*
   - *always on a diet*
   - *going for long periods of time without eating or eating as little as possible to keep weight under control*

   ### Abnormal exercise *qualities*
   - *exercising when ill or exhausted*
   - *disliking your body and feeling uncomfortable with it*
   - *exercising to punish yourself for eating*
   - *rigid exercise to lose weight or inches*
   - *exercising more than an hour a day, more than 5 times a week*
   - *feeling guilty and anxious if you don't exercise*
   - *rigidly counting miles run, pounds lifted, etc—pushing yourself to the extreme, causing physical pain, exhaustion, or injury*
   - *always on a rigid fitness program*
   - *never exercising*

   ### Abnormal eating *and* abnormal exercise
   - *extreme instead of moderate patterns*
   - *rigid, inflexible patterns*
   - *driven by negative beliefs, attitudes, and emotions*
   - *harmful consequences for personal health*
   - *moralistic judgmental attitude*

5. Summarize the themes of unhealthy patterns of eating and exercise: black and white thinking (all or nothing); rigidity; pain-inducing (physical, psychological); extreme rather than balanced; driven by negative emotions (guilt, fear, shame) instead of positive ones (self-acceptance, pleasure, pride).

6. Talk about ideal patterns of eating and exercising in a chalktalk and present an acronym for ideal patterns that will SATISFY.

● **Ideal is not much different than normal** when it comes to exercising and eating. If we could develop normal patterns, instead of the abnormal patterns that are widespread in our weight- and body-obsessed society, we would be much healthier.

● **Ideal patterns of eating and movement will satisfy you.** The characteristics of ideal patterns of eating and exercising are summarized in the acronym **SATISFY: S** = Selfish, **A** = Affirming, **T** = Thoughtful, **I** = Intuitive, **S** = Sensory, **F** = Fun, and **Y** = Yes (by all means, take care of yourself).

  ☞ *Write the acronym down the left side of a piece of newsprint. Write the corresponding word to the right of each letter.*

○ **S = Selfish.** Ideal eating and exercising is selfish. You do it for yourself, to sustain and nourish yourself, to feed and condition your body, to give yourself pleasure and satisfaction, to make your own choices, and to be responsible for yourself, your health, and your life. You do it to survive and thrive, and no one else can do it for you.

○ **A = Affirming.** Eating and exercising, in their purest form, are affirmations of life. They are existential acts that affirm your right to exist, to take up space, to move through life as a worthwhile human being.

○ **T = Thoughtful.** Ideal eating and exercise are thoughtful in that you give consideration to what is good for you, what will provide you with the best results in terms of sustenance, energy, and well-being. It takes into account your values, spiritual beliefs, lifestyle, and resources at a particular point in time.

○ **I = Intuitive.** Ideal patterns of eating and exercise are based on intuition and trust in yourself to know what you need. If you trust your intuition, you will naturally make food choices that satisfy biological and psychological needs, and you will gravitate toward exercise you love. Some people take joy in dancing, others in running, and others in biking, bowling, or weed-whacking.

© 1996 WHOLE PERSON PRESS 210 WEST MICHIGAN DULUTH MN 55802 ■ (800) 247-6789

○ **S = Sensory.** Eating and exercising are sensory experiences, and ideal patterns involve a heightened sensory awareness of hunger, fullness, satisfaction, tension, relaxation, exhilaration, pain, fatigue, and other bodily responses to food and exercise. Only by listening to your body can you care for yourself properly and give yourself the pleasure you seek.

○ **F = Fun.** Eating and exercise should be fun. Pleasure—not pain— is ideal. Enjoyment, laughter, play, optimism are all associated with ideal wellness and longevity.

○ **Y = Yes,** by all means, take care of yourself. It is good to satisfy yourself, normally and naturally, with food and exercise.

7. Invite participants to reflect on their own patterns of eating and exercise. Hand out a blank sheet of paper to each participant. Instruct them to fold it into quarters and label the four sections: **Unhealthy patterns to watch or tolerate; Unhealthy patterns to change; Healthy patterns to maintain; Healthier patterns to adopt.**

8. Provide guidelines for reflection.

➤ Look over the list of normal and abnormal eating and exercise patterns, and the acronym SATISFY. Think about your own patterns.

➤ In the **Unhealthy patterns to watch or tolerate** section, write down any eating or exercise patterns that are of concern to you but not disturbing or uncomfortable enough to warrant changing at this time.

  ➤ Are you developing a pattern of snacking when lonely and then doing more exercise to compensate the next day? Have you been exercising less, recently, or eating more fat in your diet?

➤ In the **Unhealthy patterns to change** category, write down any eating or exercise patterns you think are harmful to you, physically or psychologically.

  ➤ Are you bingeing and purging—and developing medical complications as a result? Are you becoming a couch potato? Eating more than you need to satisfy hunger?

➤ In the **Healthy patterns to maintain** category, write down the healthy eating and exercise habits you already have and want to keep doing.

  ➤ Are you walking regularly? Minimizing red meat? Are you eating nutritious foods yet allowing yourself the pleasure of other foods you love that may be less healthy?

➤ In the **Healthier patterns to adopt** section, write your ideas for improving on your current healthy patterns of eating and exercising. If you walk twice a week, could you increase it to four? If you're using milk in your coffee, could you switch to skim—or herbal tea with lemon?

9. Conclude with a chalktalk cautioning participants not to slip into thinking in absolutes about either abnormal/normal or unhealthy/ healthy.

● **Normal and healthy are fluid, flexible terms.** They cover a wide range of behavior over a period of time. Health is a dynamic, ever-changing process. Most of us move in and out of normal, abnormal, and ideal patterns. We are usually a mixture of healthy and unhealthy habits.

● **Think of yourself as *in process*.** You are evolving new patterns while you seek to maintain healthy old patterns and let go of or modify unhealthy ones. Respect and appreciate yourself as you work on this fascinating personal evolution.

● **Remember the distortions of normal in our culture.** In America, what we define as normal for weight and body appearance is not really normal. For example, Miss America contestants and *Playboy* centerfold models average *19 percent below normal weight,* which puts them in eating-disorder range. This is considered normal size for models. In our society, you may be seen as abnormal if you practice normal eating and exercising. Seek support for challenging these distorted norms and values with your words or actions.

FOR ONGOING GROUPS

■ The **Ideal Patterns** reflection is a generic process that can be easily adapted for a variety of other issues or topics such as relationships, self-care, body image, work patterns, creativity habits, etc.

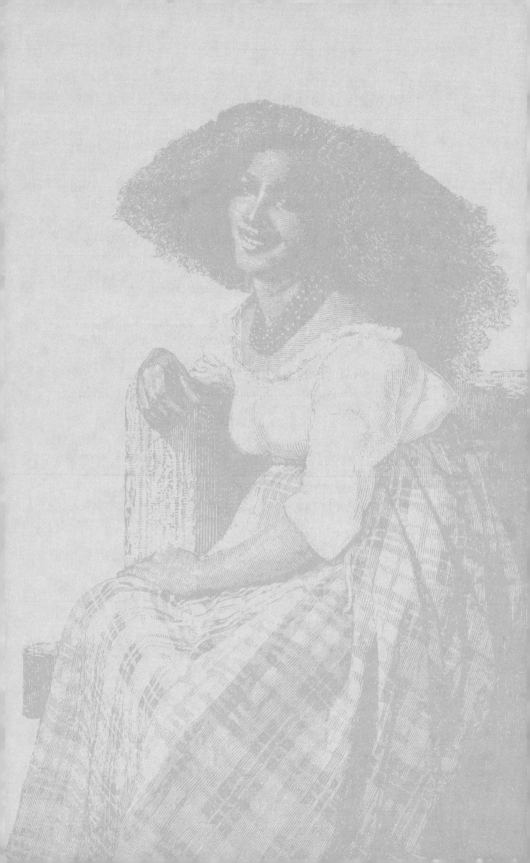

FOCUS ON

BODY IMAGE & MOVEMENT

Exercises in this section will help participants to explore personal body image from many perspectives: enjoyable movement, positive and negative attitudes and beliefs about body, historical roots of these body beliefs, and deeper connections to the inner self.

17 BODY PARTS

In this threefold exercise, participants examine themselves from head to foot, identify their most and least favorite body parts, and explore ways to develop an appreciation for undervalued body parts.

GOALS

To explore positive and negative body beliefs and attitudes.

To practice changing negative body beliefs to more positive ones.

GROUP SIZE

Unlimited.

TIME FRAME

30–40 minutes.

MATERIALS NEEDED

Body Parts worksheets, duplicated on both sides; newsprint and marker; crayons.

PROCESS

1. Invite participants to pair up (or form trios) with someone else who has a similar eye color. When everyone has partners, give guidelines for introductions.

   ➤ Close your eyes a moment and think about the part of your body that you like best.

   ➤ Open your eyes and introduce yourself to your partner(s) by telling your name, your favorite body part, and briefly explain why you like this part of your body the most.

2. Solicit examples of favorite body parts from different groups.

3. Define body image and its effect on self-esteem in a chalktalk.

   ● **Body image is very personal and subjective.** It is a picture of your body seen through your mind's eye, including *visual* (what you see in the mirror), *mental* (what you think about what you see), and *kinesthetic* (how you move through space) elements. A short, small person who moves freely may *feel* taller than a tall person who constricts her movements. A large person who sees herself as loved by many people may describe herself as huggable, lovable, and beautiful. A depressed person will usually see herself as less attractive.

● **Most people have negative body images.** In her book *Body Love,* Dr. Rita Freedman cites data indicating females of all ages are particularly dissatisfied with their bodies. One study of ten-year-old girls found that the majority saw themselves as the least attractive girl in the class. Most adult women believe they are heavier than they are or than men prefer. Less than half of adult females will say, "I like my looks the way they are."

4. Distribute **Body Parts** worksheets and crayons to each person. Invite participants to explore their body images in a graphic experiment.

➤ Imagine that the outline of a person on the worksheet represents your body.

➤ Scan the body from head to toe, considering whether you like or dislike each part of your own body.

➤ Using whatever colors, words, and symbols seem appropriate, identify those parts of your body you don't particularly like.

➤ Don't forget about small body parts such as earlobes, toes, fingernails, kneecaps, etc.

➤ Don't forget about your backside! Turn the worksheet over to mark those unlikable body parts visible from the rearview.

➤ Exchange crayons with a neighbor if you need to.

☞ *Allow 4-5 minutes for embellishing the drawing, prompting as needed to encourage detailed and specific assessments.*

5. After 3–5 minutes, make a large body outline on newsprint for recording the group's judgments. Work down the body from head to toe, asking at each body part if there is any participant who does not like that part of her body. Include hair, forehead, eyebrows, eyes, nose, cheeks, mouth, ears, chin, neck, shoulders, arms, hands, fingers, breasts/chest, abdomen, waist, back, shoulders, buttocks, hips, thighs, knees, calves, ankles, feet, toes.

For each body part judged unsatisfactory by *anyone,* color that area of the large body poster.

6. Summarize the results of the group poll and comment on typical gender differences in body image.

● **Typically, men are less critical of their bodies;** women are more critical of theirs. Men see their bodies as fine; women are cruel in their talk about their own and other women's bodies. Men treat body flaws as human; women are deadly serious.

- **Men like to take up lots of space;** women like to take up as little space as possible. Men generally underestimate their body size; women overestimate their body size. Men focus on face; women focus on body.
- **Men are more internally focused;** women are more externally focused for a sense of self.

7. Introduce the idea that body image can be changed.

- **Negative body beliefs are just that—beliefs.** And beliefs are changeable. They are nothing more than what we tell ourselves.
- **You can choose to believe differently.** You can decide to think of your long nose as interesting, as giving you character. You can choose to believe that your large body is truly magnificent. Whatever you decide will become your reality.

8. Invite participants to explore one of their negative body beliefs in more depth.

➤ Look over your drawing again and think about each of the parts of your body you do not like.

➤ Select your *least favorite* body part and write it at the top of the list under the **Old Beliefs** section of your worksheet.

   ➤ List all of the reasons why you don't like this body part.

   ➤ What are your beliefs and attitudes about this body part? Do you believe it is ugly, defective, or a symbol of personal failure? Do you see it as an object for ridicule, rejection, or exploitation?

     ☞ *Pause here, and after each group of instructions, to allow participants time to reflect and write.*

➤ Now try to look at this disliked body part with new eyes.

   ➤ What positive characteristic does it have?

   ➤ How has it served you over the years?

   ➤ What pleasant memories or sensations do you associate with this body part?

   ➤ How would a person who loved you describe this body part?

   ➤ Write a list of positive things about this body part in the **New Beliefs** section.

➤ Now assume you will adopt these new beliefs.

   ➤ What *actions* will you take to live out these new beliefs and show appreciation, respect, and enjoyment of this body part (eg, wear shorts, get a pedicure, go dancing, dress to size)? Record them in the **Actions** section.

9. Invite participants to share their pictures and plans for change.

> ➤ Share some or all of your drawing with your partner(s) and briefly explain why you do not like these parts of your body.

>> ☞ *Be aware that some participants may feel exposed and vulnerable when asked to share their drawings. Make it clear that it is okay to remain private by sharing only select portions or passing altogether on their turn to share.*

> ➤ Each person has 1 minute to share.

> ➤ The person with the brightest crayon is appointed timekeeper.

10. Solicit examples of plans for changing negative body beliefs to positive ones.

11. Conclude with a chalktalk encouraging participants to work on liking all their body parts.

> ● **Find reasons to like all your body parts.** You are a whole person and will feel happier and healthier when you value all of your body parts unconditionally, simply because they are part of you.

> ● **Proceed with caution and care.** It is not easy to change old, internalized beliefs. You may have to confront or challenge old family messages, societal and cultural stereotypes of how you should look, or past hurts or traumas associated with certain parts of your body. Make sure you have people who will support you in this process, especially if you have been a victim of abuse or neglect.

> ● **Be patient.** Your beliefs, attitudes, and feelings *will* change, provided that you persist in living out attitudes of respect, appreciation, and enjoyment of your body.

FOR ONGOING GROUPS

> ■ This exercise can be used early in the group process as a tool for assessing body image problems, or as a catalyst for goal-setting. It can also be used as follow-up near the end of the course or group sessions to see how perceptions of body image have changed or have been influenced by the group learning experience.

The body-coloring process was contributed by Laura Field, who adapted it from an original process by Gail Johnston. The body beliefs portion was contributed by Lucia Capacchione.

BODY PARTS

OLD BELIEFS
I don't like my ——————————— (body part)
because I believe it is . . .

NEW BELIEFS
The positive things about this part of my body are . . .

ACTIONS
To celebrate, appreciate, and enjoy this part of my body,
I will . . .

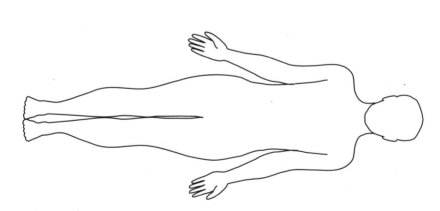

18 FINDING CENTER

In this soothing meditation, participants find the sacred, centering places in their body.

GOALS

To affirm friendly connections with the body and identify personal centers of energy, wisdom, and balance.

To learn centering as a skill for managing stress.

GROUP SIZE

Unlimited.

TIME FRAME

20–30 minutes.

MATERIALS NEEDED

Finding My Center script; CD or cassette player and slow, flowing relaxation music (optional); newsprint; marker.

PROCESS

1. Start with a chalktalk about the power of centering.

   ● **Everyone has a center in her body.** This is the place of balance and harmony within yourself. It is the home of your life force, the center of your being or spirit. It is the temple of your inner wisdom, your truest self, your heart and soul.

   ● **It is easy to become disconnected from our centers.** So many things can throw us off balance:

      ○ **Childhood abuse.** If a person in power took control of your life, wouldn't allow you to speak up for yourself, or made you live in ways that violate your deepest beliefs about yourself and the world, you may have learned to disconnect from yourself as a survival mechanism.

      ○ **Eating disorders.** If food, body weight, and body image have become the focus of your attention, you may have lost touch with your inner self. Obsessive thinking keeps the focus on external, not internal, ways of being.

      ○ **Other addictions.** Alcohol and drug abuse, gambling, spending, shopping, work, and many other addictions can keep you from yourself because you become preoccupied with the addictive substance, which becomes the center of your life. The insidious process of addiction may cause you to abandon everything that is important to you.

○ **Denial of feelings.** When you discount, disregard, or deny your feelings, you lose trust in yourself and your body's natural rhythm. It's easy to lose the inner direction that is supplied by feeling and intuition.

○ **Ongoing stress and overly busy lives.** If you are so busy coping with day-to-day stress that you don't take time for quiet reflection, you deny yourself the nourishment, relaxation, and reassurance that could come from finding your calm center in the midst of the storm.

2. Briefly explain the process of meditation and announce that everyone will have the opportunity to participate in a meditation for finding personal center.

● **Meditation is a natural way of restoring balance.** It involves stopping what you are doing at any given moment, allowing yourself a few minutes of uninterrupted quiet time, relaxing through deep breathing, and concentrating on a selected image, thought, or sound.

● **Everyone knows how to relax.** Whenever you've given yourself *staring time* at the beach, solitary walks through the woods, engrossing music at a concert, or private prayers, you have probably meditated. Such times of contemplation provide solid anchors during less peaceful moments.

3. Answer questions participants may have about meditation and then prepare everyone for a short guided meditation.

➤ Make yourself as comfortable as possible, sitting in your chair or on the floor.

➣ Remove glasses, shoes, or any other uncomfortable accessory.

➤ Relax and follow along with the script.

4. Dim the lights, play soft, flowing background music, and slowly read the **Finding My Center** script.

5. Allow a moment or two for reentry, then encourage participants to stretch briefly. Invite participants to share what they've learned.

➤ Remain standing and, without talking, put your hand on your favorite center spot in your body.

> ➤ Keeping your hand on this spot, silently move around the room and allow others to see your center while you observe theirs.
> ➤ Still without talking, pair up with another person whose center is the same or similar to yours.
> ➤ Decide who will be ***Body*** and who will be ***Soul***.
>> ➤ ***Body*** goes first. Take 2 minutes to talk about your discoveries during the guided mediation.
>> ➤ ***Soul*** listens attentively, without interruption.
>> ➤ After 2 minutes, reverse roles so ***Soul*** can talk while ***Body*** listens.

6. Invite feedback from participants about their centering experiences. Address any questions or issues raised and then conclude with a chalktalk about the use of meditation as a tool for staying centered.

   ● **Practice mini-meditations everyday.** No matter where you are or what you are doing, take time to stop, take a deep breath, focus on your center, and calm yourself. Try putting your hand on your center, closing your eyes and saying to yourself:

   I am connected to my center.   *I listen to myself.*
   I am at home with myself.   *I am restoring my balance.*
   I take time to center myself.

   ● **Develop meditation skills.** Read a book (eg, *Inquire Within* by Andrew Schwartz, *Working Inside Out* by Margo Adair, or *Complete Meditation* by Steve Kravette) or take a class in meditation. Practice by setting aside a longer period of time (twenty minutes or more) every day when you can meditate without interruption.

   ● **Trust your instincts.** If your heart longs for music, play music. If your body yearns to move, walk or dance when meditating. If your spirit wants to sing, go ahead and sing. If you need to hear your own voice, try a mantra or phrase you repeat over and over. If you want to be in water, try meditating in a hot bath or at the lake. Do whatever it takes to center yourself.

   ● **Make meditation a way of life,** not just a daily routine. Learn to live consistently from the center of your being—your truest self.

FOR ONGOING GROUPS

   ■ Try starting or ending the group with a short meditation. This is a powerful way to intensify energy in the group. It also sends the message to group members that taking time to center yourself is a valued and worthwhile use of time.

FINDING MY CENTER Script

Allow yourself time to become quiet now . . .
and turn your attention inward . . .
Let your thoughts drift away . . . like clouds . . .
softly scooting across the sky . . .

Take a deep breath . . . and exhale slowly . . .
letting tension leave your body . . .
and drift away . . . with the wind . . .
leaving you relaxed . . . and quiet . . .
focused on your breathing . . .
hearing yourself breathe in deeply . . .
and out again . . . with a sigh . . .

☞ *Pause 5 seconds*

Allow yourself to stay focused on this moment . . .
If your mind wanders . . . simply notice it happening . . .
and gently pull your attention back . . .
to this time with yourself . . .
and the rhythm of your breathing . . .

☞ *Pause 5 seconds*

Imagine that your soul exists somewhere in your body . . .
Where would it be? . . .
Allow yourself to find this place . . .
and gently touch this place now . . .
Allow your hand to stroke this spot . . .
and connect with it . . .

☞ *Pause 10 seconds*

Imagine that your body is a building . . .
In one room of this building . . .
there is a spot where you would feel most relaxed . . . and at home . . .
Find this place now . . . and notice where it is located . . .
Touch the outward location for this space . . . on your body . . .
giving yourself a gentle reminder . . . of where to find your internal home . . .

Now pretend that you are going to balance your physical body on a fulcrum . . .
Where is the point of contact . . . on which you will balance?
Touch this spot now . . .
with gentleness and care . . .
acknowledging this place of balance for your body . . .

Take a few slow and very deep breaths . . .
Where does your breath originate? . . .

Take another very deep breath . . .
Where does the deepest breath reach? . . .
Touch these places now . . .
and gently pat . . . this center of your life force . . .

Using you inner voice . . .
say "I am me" several times . . .
as you point to yourself . . .
Where do you point? . . .
Which place feels trust? . . .
Touch the place that is you . . .
and gently stroke this spot . . .
the center of your being . . .

Notice that you may have several centers . . .
they are all valid . . . and true for you . . .
Perhaps you have a favorite . . .
Take time now to select the one . . .
that feels best to you . . .
Trust yourself to choose the space . . .
where you can be yourself . . .
know yourself . . .
and love yourself . . .

Trust yourself to find the center . . .
that holds your truth . . . and your wisdom . . .
the source of your light . . . and energy . . .
and life.

Keep your hand on this special place . . .
while you prepare to return to your surroundings . . .
secure in knowing . . .
that you can find this place again . . .
anytime . . . anywhere . . .
when you need it . . .

When you are ready . . .
slowly turn your attention to the room
and rejoin the group . . .
feeling centered . . .
with yourself and others in the room . . .
maintaining the balance you found . . .
in your body.

Finding My Center *script was adapted from* **Wellness: Small Changes You Can Use to Make a Big Difference** *(Berkeley CA: Ten Speed Press, 1991) by Regina Sara Ryan and John Travis.*

19 MIRROR, MIRROR

This simple exercise is a profound reminder that attitude toward self is far more important than physical beauty.

GOALS

To explore the relationship of fairness and self-esteem.

To recognize personal choices for being fair with oneself.

GROUP SIZE

Unlimited.

TIME FRAME

30–45 minutes.

MATERIALS NEEDED

Mirror, Mirror worksheets; small hand or pocket mirrors for each participant; newsprint or poster; marker; masking tape.

PROCESS

1. Set the stage for this exercise with a chalktalk about self-esteem and fairness.

    ● **Most people don't like what they see in the mirror.** In the fairy tale *Snow White and the Seven Dwarfs,* the wicked witch looks into her magic mirror and says: "Mirror, mirror, on the wall, who's the fairest of them all?" She wants to be the most beautiful. We're no different from the witch. Every time we look into the mirror we're making comparisons, hoping what we see reflected back will measure up to some hypothetical standard of perfection—beauty, talent, strength, wit, charm—like the witch, we are usually disappointed. And we imagine the rest of the world is too.

    ● **Fairy tales aren't real.** If you follow this fairy tale pattern, you aren't truly being *fair* to yourself. Instead of judging yourself with compassion and fairness, you judge yourself harshly, focus on your shortcomings, minimize your achievements, and discount your personal beauty. You may be generous with praise, love, appreciation, acceptance, patience, tolerance, and forgiveness for others, but withhold these same gifts from yourself. Why continue this fairy tale route to low self-esteem?

● **Family is our first and most powerful mirror—and shaper of self-esteem.** Some families are able to provide the loving, nurturing experiences that foster self-esteem; other families cannot give the consistent support or care needed for children to grow into adults with a positive self-image. Four key variables of family life influence our esteem.

○ **Atmosphere.** We all need emotional support, but not everyone gets it. Some families focus on what you are doing wrong and what needs to be corrected, instead of how important and lovable you are. In these families there is little or no affirmation for *being,* because the focus is on *doing*—and doing it right! That's not fair!

○ **Mistakes.** Everyone makes mistakes. Healthy families recognize this fact. They hold people accountable, help others learn from their mistakes, forgive wrongdoing, and move on. Other families do not forgive mistakes. Instead of problem solving, these families get stuck on the problem and cannot move beyond it. As a result, people end up feeling perpetually bad about themselves. That's not fair!

○ **Pain.** When people are physically or emotionally hurt, they need care and comfort. Many families can provide this nurturing and seem to have an endless capacity for love, empathy, hugs, and listening. Other families have trouble giving this vital nourishment. They may respond to a child's tears with anger, punishment, shaming, withdrawal, rejection, or abuse. This sends the message that it is bad to be needy and you are unworthy of kindness. That's not fair!

○ **Expectations.** Families should help their members achieve their goals. This can be done by having flexible, humane, and age-appropriate rules. If perfection is expected, family members will fail no matter what they do. This system erodes the esteem of its members. That's not fair!

● **For healthier self-esteem be fair with yourself.** Start by exploring the ways you learned to be unfair with yourself in the past, then discover new strategies for making more honest and positive appraisals in the future.

2. Hand out **Mirror, Mirror** worksheets and guide participants through a reflection on the nature of their own childhood family environment.

☞ *Solicit childhood examples of each type as you work through the four categories.*

➤ Direct your attention to the upper half of your mirror that is labeled **Childhood.**

➤ What was your family atmosphere like? Was it harsh and critical, or permissive and supportive? Did your parents encourage you or put you down?

   ➤ Estimate the percentage of time your family was *supportive* and the percentage of time they were *critical*. The total should add up to 100%.

   ➤ Record these percentages in the section for **Childhood Family Atmosphere.**

   ➤ Add one or two examples of the ways your family showed support or indicated criticism (eg, telling you how capable you were, letting you solve problems and make mistakes, or telling you you weren't capable, taking over, doing everything for you).

➤ How were mistakes handled in your family? Were you held accountable, given the chance to learn from your errors, and forgiven? Or were you continually reminded of your mistakes?

   ➤ Estimate the proportion of times you were *forgiven* and the proportion of times you were *reminded of your mistakes*.

   ➤ Write these percentages in the section for **Childhood Mistakes.**

   ➤ Write down one or two examples of how you were forgiven or reminded of your mistakes (eg, given a hug and kiss from parents after you apologized for a mistake, or treated to a week of rejecting silence from a parent following an argument).

➤ How did people in your family react when you were hurting? Did they respond with care and concern, or ridicule and rejection?

   ➤ Estimate the percentage of time you *received comfort* and the percentage of time you were *rejected*.

   ➤ Write these percentages in the **Childhood Pain** section.

   ➤ Write one or two examples of how you were comforted or rejected (eg, parents holding you and letting you cry, or calling you a crybaby and sending you to your room when you were upset).

➤ How would you describe the expectations your family had of you? Were they flexible and humane, or rigid and inhumane?

   ➤ Estimate the proportion of family rules that were *flexible and humane* and those that were *rigid and inhumane*.

   ➤ Write these percentages in the section for **Childhood Expectations.**

© 1996 WHOLE PERSON PRESS 210 WEST MICHIGAN DULUTH MN 55802 ■(800) 247-6789

➤ Write one or two examples of flexible, humane rules or rigid, inhumane rules in your family (eg, everyone shared chores and your responsibility was clearly defined as doing supper dishes, or you were expected to do all the housework and keep the house spotless when you were ten years old).

3. Interrupt the personal reflection process and poll the group to see how many felt that their family atmosphere, rules, expectations, and ways of handling mistakes and pain were fair and humane? Weave responses into a chalktalk on fairness.

● **Dysfunctional families have distorted views of what's fair or appropriate.** When we grow up in such a family, it is very hard to know what is reasonable, fair, and humane, since the norm in our family is unfair.

● **Fairness implies the absence of injustice.** One party is not favored over another. Instead, all people are put on an equal footing. Fairness means the rules of a game or a family are followed with honesty and consistency.

4. Pass out mirrors to participants and explain that we will not be focusing on fairness as *beauty*, but on fairness as *justice* and *humane treatment*. Invite participants to reflect upon their *fairness with themselves*.

➤ Look into the mirror and say, "Mirror, mirror on the wall, who's the *fairest* of them all?"

  ➤ Think in terms of being *fair* with yourself rather than beauty.

  ➤ Are you permissive and supportive of yourself, or harsh and critical?

  ➤ When you make a mistake, do you accept and forgive yourself, or shame and blame yourself?

  ➤ When you are hurting do you give yourself or ask others for support and comfort, or do you isolate yourself and suffer in silence?

  ➤ Are your personal expectations of yourself realistic and flexible, or unreasonable and rigid?

5. Allow 2 minutes for quiet reflection and then ask participants to complete the bottom half of their **Mirror, Mirror** worksheet.

➤ Consider the four categories of fairness for your **Adult Life**, recording percentages and examples as you did in the **Childhood** sections.

  ➤ Think in terms of being fair with yourself rather than beauty.

  ➤ Are you permissive and supportive of yourself, or harsh and critical?

➤ When you make a mistake, do you accept and forgive yourself, or get stuck on your mistakes?

➤ When you are hurting do you give yourself or ask others for support and comfort, or do you isolate yourself and suffer in silence?

➤ Are your personal expectations of yourself realistic and flexible, or unreasonable and rigid?

6. When participants have completed their worksheets, suggest a process for further reflection.

➤ Observe the difference between your **Childhood** and **Adult Life** mirrors. Do you notice any changes, or are you repeating your childhood experiences in your present day life?

➤ Jot down your insights at the bottom of the page in the space for **Reflections.**

7. Poll the group on their responses to the issue of fairness.

✔ How many believe you are being fair with yourself?

✔ How many discovered that you are living out childhood standards of fairness in your adult life?

8. Point out that regardless of childhood learning, participants can learn to be more fair and affirming of themselves. Invite participants to brainstorm a list of affirming ideas or statements that might help them to be more fair with themselves. Write all examples on a poster or newsprint, and hang it on the wall.

☞ *Offer some examples to get the ball rolling.*
  I love me, I love myself.
  I accept myself as I am.
  I will be fair with myself.
  It is okay to make mistakes.
  I deserve care and comfort when I am hurting.
  It's okay to ask for help when I need it.
  I set reasonable goals for myself.
  I support and affirm myself.

9. Invite participants to try out these new attitudes of fairness, using a litany of affirmations done with a partner.

➤ Locate your small mirror and have it ready for use in the litany.

➤ Pair up with someone you do not know well.

➤ Decide who will be *Snow White* and who will be the **Queen.**

➣ **Queens** go first. Select an affirmation from the list and read it, while looking into your mirror.

➣ **Snow Whites** respond by looking into your own mirror and repeating the **Queen's** affirmation out loud.

➤ **Snow Whites** then select an affirmation from the list, read it while looking into your own mirror, and **Queens** respond by repeating the affirmation while looking into your mirror.

➤ Alternate between reader and responder, until several new attitudes have been practiced, then talk about what it was like to state your affirmations out loud with a partner.

➤ Each person has 2 minutes to share her response to the exercise.

10. After 5–8 minutes, interrupt the small group discussions and solicit feedback from participants about this exercise. Weave participants' responses into a chalktalk on ways to become more fair with yourself.

● **Be tolerant of uncomfortable feelings** when you try to become more fair with yourself. If this is new for you, you can expect to feel anxious, guilty, embarrassed, ashamed, or foolish when you affirm yourself by words or deeds.

● **Be patient with yourself** as you try to change. Go slowly, accept yourself where you are, seek the support you need.

● **Be bold** in your use of the mirror. Tell yourself wonderful things. Then act as if you believe them. Eventually you will.

● **Be honest.** Look into the mirror and ask, "Mirror, mirror on the wall, who's the fairest of them all?" If you're not being fair with yourself, remind yourself of your human rights and give them to yourself.

FOR ONGOING GROUPS

▦ Make mirror work a routine part of your sessions. If possible, keep a full-length mirror in the group room. Have participants stand in front of the mirror and describe what they see. Invite other group members to give a reality check by describing what they see, especially the positive attributes the person in front of the mirror has missed.

▦ Assign mirror work as homework including the affirmations practiced in this exercise. Incorporate participants' experiences into ongoing group process.

This exercise was contributed by Dick Boyum.

MIRROR, MIRROR

CHILDHOOD

FAMILY ATMOSPHERE
supportive / critical

MISTAKES
*accountability & forgiveness /
stuck on mistakes*

PAIN
comfort / rejection

EXPECTATIONS
*flexible & humane /
rigid & inhumane*

ADULT LIFE

FAMILY ATMOSPHERE
supportive / critical

MISTAKES
*accountability & forgiveness /
stuck on mistakes*

PAIN
comfort / rejection

EXPECTATIONS
*flexible & humane /
rigid & inhumane*

REFLECTIONS: _____

_____

_____

_____

_____

_____

20 MOVING ATTITUDES

In this powerful exercise, participants explore the way body attitudes affect body image and the way we move through life.

GOALS

To identify how negative body beliefs affect movement, posture, and body tension.

To try on new beliefs.

GROUP SIZE

Unlimited.

TIME FRAME

45 minutes.

MATERIALS NEEDED

Moving Attitudes worksheet; spacious, comfortable room free of obstructions.

PROCESS

1. Set the stage for this exercise with a chalktalk about mind/body communication.

   ● **Your body is a powerful, expressive instrument.** It communicates your innermost feelings and attitudes to the outside world. Have you ever sat in an airport terminal and watched people as they walk by? There are those who charge ahead with determination, those who meander along, daydreaming, those who appear shy and unsure, those who seem like bold peacocks displaying their feathers to the world. Every person has a personal style, a unique way of being in her body and moving through life.

   ● **Mind/body communication is circular.** Your mind affects your body and your body in turn affects your mind. Your attitudes translate into body patterns that become chronic and in turn color your experience of being in the world. If your attitude is body shame, you may hold your body in a slouch or slump, unconsciously trying to be less visible to the world. This inward pulling will affect you physiologically, psychologically, and socially. You may feel tense and sore in your body, depressed in mental outlook, and withdrawn or isolated in social relationships.

● **Most mind/body communication is unconscious.** We are not aware of our body attitudes until we make them conscious. As your self-awareness grows, you can make intentional decisions to change your body language, body image, and way of moving in the world.

2. Explain that the purpose of this session is for participants to explore their own mind/body interactions. Hand out **Moving Attitudes** worksheets and instruct participants to reflect on their negative body attitudes.

➤ Turn your attention to **Question 1** on your worksheet.

➤ Take a moment and write down three of your most chronic *negative attitudes* about your body. These are the beliefs, feelings, or attitudes that you are convinced are *true* statements about your body.

☞ *Solicit examples from participants to stimulate ideas (eg, I'm not good enough; I'm fat; I'm ugly).*

➤ Now circle or star the statement that reflects your *most central negative attitude* toward yourself.

3. Instruct participants to set down their worksheets for a moment, and then guide them through an exploration of body image through movement.

☞ *The movement sequence should take 2-3 minutes. Be sure people keep moving throughout.*

Stand up, close your eyes, take some full breaths, and go into your body . . .
Get in touch with the way you are feeling about it right now . . .
Open your eyes and begin to walk around . . .
As you continue to walk around, reflect on these questions:

☞ *Pause after each question to allow time for reflection. Make sure participants keep walking while they do this reflection.*

What does your body say by the way it moves through space?
What is your body language telling others about how you feel about yourself?
What attitudes are you projecting by the way you move?
The way you carry yourself?
The expression on your face?
By your willingness to make eye contact?

4. Interrupt the movement and ask participants to return to their home base and worksheet. Note that people should consider this movement experience as their *usual movement,* or normal way of moving.

➤ Answer **Question 2** on your worksheet.

➤ What are you projecting in the way you carry yourself, move, use body language, etc? In other words, what are you saying to the world about how you feel about yourself?

➤ What kind(s) of responses do you expect from others? Are you projecting confidence, fear, curiosity, boredom? Are you feeling proud, ashamed, pleased, sad? Do you expect acceptance, rejection, affirmation, or indifference from others?

5. Invite participants to explore further how mental attitudes affect the body and body image by experimenting with another moving experience. Ask them to look back at **Question 1** and focus on their *most central negative body image* for this activity.

Stand up and walk around again in your usual, normal way . . .

Now stand still and close your eyes . . .
Bring to mind the statement you wrote down as your chronic negative attitude . . .
As if you were an actor, get into the character . . .
Try on *that attitude as if it were a cloak that you put on, and let yourself really experience what it means to be you when you identify yourself this way . . .*

Open your eyes and begin to walk around with this attitude . . .
Exaggerate it a bit to make its impact clear . . .

Continue walking and notice your response to these questions.

How are you feeling? . . .
Notice your posture, carriage, facial expression, sensations, thoughts, feelings, body tension patterns, impulses, etc.
How does it feel to be in the world when you define yourself this way?

How do you feel in relation to others?
Go up to someone and communicate the attitude with your body, and notice how it feels.

What do you like about this negative body attitude?
What don't you like about it?
How do you feel it limits you?
What does it give you permission to do . . .be . . .feel . . . or not do . . . be . . . feel?
Who would you be without this attitude?
What risk would you take if you let go of this attitude?
What might you lose if you gave it up?

6. Interrupt the movement and ask participants to sit down and write their answers to **Question 3** on the worksheet.

  ☞ *You might want to expand this section by repeating Steps 5 and 6, inviting participants to act out their second and third negative body images.*

7. Invite participants to share examples of their discoveries, raise concerns, or ask questions about the process so far. When you are satisfied that participants are moving through the process and not getting stuck or confused, move on to the next step.

8. Ask the group to brainstorm a list of new, more positive body attitudes and to express these in a short positive statement. Write these statements on newsprint.

  ☞ *Prime the pump with examples:*
  I am perfectly all right just the way I am.
  I like myself and feel easy in my body.
  This is my body, this is where I live.
  I'm good enough.
  I am a uniquely beautiful woman inside and out, and I know it.
  I am in touch with and proud of my sexuality and my womanliness.

9. Invite participants to try another kind of experience in moving attitudes, using a *positive statement of their choice* from the group list.

  ☞ *Be sure people keep moving throughout.*

  Stand up and prepare to do some more walking.
  You have just experienced how your chronic attitudes affect your being in the world. Let's see now how new attitudes could change your body and your feelings.

  Focus on one new positive attitude you'd like to experiment with . . .
  Try on *your new body attitude . . .*
  As you try it on, take a moment to let the statement register, then translate it into a way of carrying yourself and walk around as if you believe it about yourself . . .
  Now start walking and try on the new attitude . . .

  How do you feel?
  How does this new attitude translate into shifts in carriage, movement, expression, etc?
  What do you like about it? What is hard to accept about it?
  Is there anything scary about it?
  How do you imagine others will respond to you?

10. Invite people to return to their seats and answer **Question 4** on the worksheet.

   ➤ How did you react to your new attitude statement? What feelings did it bring up? What was striking or informative about your reaction?

   ➤ What did you learn about your fears and resistance to changing the way you feel about your body?

11. Invite participants to share examples of their reactions and resistances to changing body attitudes.

12. Challenge participants to create their own **moving affirmation.**

   ➤ Create a positive attitude statement that embodies the qualities you would like to have as you move through life.

   ➤ Think of a statement that your body can speak out to the world, a new message to hold in mind when thinking about your body.

   ➤ Ask your body to help you construct the affirmation. Ask your body what the body would like to hear from you so that it feels accepted and loved.

   ➤ Ask yourself what you need to believe about your bodyself right now. Frame your affirmation in the positive form, *I, _name_, am _____ (eg, a beautiful woman, growing to love my body, etc).*

   ➤ Write your affirmation on the worksheet under **Question 5.**

13. Solicit examples, then ask participants to try on their new personal **moving affirmation.**

   *Stand up, begin to walk around and **try on** your new affirmation. As you walk around, repeat your moving affirmation over and over.*

   Move around in your affirmation . . .
   *Let your body explore what it means to be **this** you . . .*
   when you believe this affirmation about yourself.
   Notice your posture, your body language,
   the way you feel in your body . . .
   the quality of your movement, your relationship to your environment,
   your body impulses, your self-image, as you move.

   Memorize these feelings and let them flow into your dominant hand (right hand if you're right-handed), locking them there. Let that hand become the repository of the feelings that this affirmation evokes and embodies for you.
   As you walk around, squeeze your hand to bring up the affirmative feeling . . . and walk around for 30 seconds embodying it . . .

   ☞ *Wait 30 seconds before giving the next instruction.*

*Now let go and walk around for 30 seconds in your **normal** mode.*

☞ *Wait 30 seconds.*

*Now alternate between **normal** and **new** when I give the signal.*
As you shift back and forth,
notice the changes in the way you take on the world.
Notice what it is like to be in the world as a person who feels this way.
For each attitude, pay attention to any resistance that comes up
as you move with your new affirmation . . . What feels risky?
What obstacles do you feel that might prevent your embracing
this attitude fully?

☞ *Give the signal to shift every 30 seconds for 2 minutes.*

14. Invite participants to write about their experiences by answering **Questions 6** and **7** on their worksheet.

15. Divide the group into small groups of 3–5 people and give suggestions for group discussion.

   ➤ Share what you learned about negative body image and your willingness to move into new body attitudes.

   ➤ Each person has 3 minutes to share.

16. Solicit examples of resistance to new, positive body attitudes, summarize common issues, and respond to questions raised by participants.

17. Conclude with a chalktalk on how participants can take their affirmations into the real world.

   ● **Practice body affirmations.** Set aside at least 15 minutes each day to move your affirmation into your real life. Try it out in different settings: at home, at work, in social situations.

   ● **Give yourself time to change.** It takes a long time to change body attitudes, and it's hard work! Pace yourself, go slowly, and celebrate the small successes as you go.

FOR ONGOING GROUPS

   ▨ This is an ideal exercise for ongoing groups. You can break the process down into several sessions and take extra time to process each part in more depth.

   ▨ This process is most appropriate for groups that have established trust and mutual support.

*This exercise was contributed by Marcia Germaine Hutchinson, EdD, author of **Transforming Body Image: Learning to Love the Body You Have** (Freedom CA: Crossing Press, 1985).*

MOVING ATTITUDES

1. Chronic Negative Body Attitudes

    a.

    b.

    c.

2. Usual Movement

    What I'm telling the world about my body . . .

    Responses I expect from others . . .

3. Most Central Negative Attitude

    I noticed . . .

    I felt . . .

    I was surprised by . . .

    If I let go of this attitude I would . . .

4. New Attitude

    I noticed . . .

    I felt . . .

    I learned . . .

5. My custom designed **moving affirmation** is . . .

6. My **moving affirmation** changed (attitudes, expectations, behaviors) . . .

7. The barriers that could stop me from adopting my **moving affirmation** are . . .

21 PHYSICAL ACTIVITY CONTINUUM

This exercise uses principles of values clarification to help participants explore their past, present, and future activity levels in a nonjudgmental manner.

GOALS

To increase understanding of how physical activity levels can change over time.

To address barriers to increasing physical activity.

GROUP SIZE

Unlimited.

TIME FRAME

45–60 minutes.

MATERIALS NEEDED

Newsprint and marker.

PROCESS

1. Introduce the topic with a short chalktalk on activity patterns.

   ● **Physical activity levels can change over time.** This depends on what else is going on in your life at any point in time. Are you in your 20s, single, and playing on two softball teams? Or are you in your 50s, raising teenagers, and working at a desk job? Are you in good physical health or struggling with a disabling illness? Does your family enjoy exercise—or prefer to play chess, read, or watch TV?

   ● **Activity changes are not good or bad.** It is not helpful to judge yourself as *good* when you are running daily or *bad* if your only activity is punching the remote control. It is helpful to simply observe your patterns and learn from them. Many of us have experienced a time when activity was enjoyable, and when we look at current activity it's helpful to get in touch with past enjoyment.

2. Ask people to imagine an invisible line drawn down the center of the room. Then set up the extremes of exercise possibilities.

   ➤ Imagine that one end of this line, or continuum, is the extreme of *Mary Marathoner!* Mary ran a marathon the first day she was born and has run a marathon every day since. *Exercise all day, every day is her motto.*

➤ Pretend that the other extreme end of the continuum is *Sally Sofa*. Sally was born on the sofa, went to school from the sofa, and has spent her whole life sitting on the sofa. Her motto is *No exercise at all for me.*

☞ *Point out that obviously, no one is this extreme. These are exaggerated examples for purposes of the exercise.*

3. Invite participants to place themselves on the continuum.

➤ Think back to when you were about *nine years old*, remembering how active you were at this time of your life.

➤ Stand up and move to a place on the continuum that best represents how active you were when you were *nine years old.*

☞ *Remind participants that it is unlikely that anyone will be at either extreme of the continuum, and to find a place that best represents their level of activity.*

4. When all have a place on the continuum, ask them to share stories with a neighbor.

➤ Talk to a person near you about your activity level when you were nine.

➤ Describe how active you were and what you were doing.

➤ Tell what you liked about what you were doing.

➤ Talk about what helped or hindered your level of activity.

5. After 2–4 minutes, guide participants to explore another time in their activity history.

➤ Close your eyes and focus again on what you said about your activity at age nine.

➤ Now move ahead in your life to when you were *sixteen years old.*

➤ Open your eyes and once again take a position on the continuum that represents your level of activity at *age sixteen.*

☞ *Most people will move at least a bit.*

➤ Once again talk with a different neighbor about your activity at age sixteen, what you liked about what you were doing, and what helped or hindered your level of activity.

6. Repeat the activity continuum process for one or two more ages, tailoring your choices to the group (eg, early 20s, early 30s, middle age, five years ago, etc).

7. At each age solicit examples of activities people have enjoyed.

8. As a final exploration, ask participants to consider present and future activity levels.

   ➤ Now move to the place on the continuum that represents *how active you are now.*

   ➢ Describe your activity level with a new neighbor.

   ➤ Move to the place that represents *how active you would really like to be.* What is a realistic goal for you now?

   ➢ As you describe your desired activity levels to a neighbor, also talk about what barriers you might encounter in reaching that goal.

9. Invite participants to return to their seats. Solicit examples of the main barriers to activity people encounter in the present or anticipate in the future. As barriers are identified, list them on newsprint and ask for advice from other participants who have experienced some success in overcoming that barrier. Record these suggestions on a separate newsprint.

10. Lead the group in a brainstorming session to identify additional strategies for overcoming common barriers to a more active lifestyle.

    ☞ For instance, **no time** *could be handled by breaking activity into small, do-able, ten-minute segments, or scheduling activity time into every day.*

11. Summarize the discussion with a chalktalk encouraging participants to take steps toward their activity goals.

    ● **There is no right or wrong activity pattern.** Everyone's experience is different. Awareness of your unique history and activity pattern is the first step in making changes.

    ● **Recall past pleasures of physical activity.** While you may not be able to return to that exact activity, you can perhaps now include some elements of that pleasure. For instance, if you liked dancing with your friends as a teenager, you can crank up the stereo and dance at home as a warm-up to going out dancing with friends. If you liked jumping rope, enroll in a Jump for Your Heart fund-raiser or find other like-minded folks who might join you for Double Dutch.

    ● **Barriers are not excuses.** Calling barriers *excuses* minimizes the reality of how difficult it is to increase physical activity. It is more helpful to validate barriers and then work to remove them.

● **It is normal to move up and down a continuum of activity** at different times of our lives. If we've moved in the past, we can move again. But we need to have patience with ourselves and take small steps toward our goal.

FOR ONGOING GROUPS

This process is easily adaptable. Try the continuum for exploration of a variety of themes and issues: body image, relationship with food, self-esteem, size-acceptance, etc.

This exercise was contributed by Pat Lyons, coauthor of **Great Shape: The First Fitness Guide for Large Women** *(Palo Alto CA: Bull Publishing, 1988), who credits Syd Simon for devising the original values continuum.*

22 SENSUAL WALK

Participants take a walk outdoors and indoors to explore the ways physical senses impact body/mind health.

GOALS

To discover how the physical senses affect body/mind health.

To enjoy the benefits of exercise and movement.

GROUP SIZE

Unlimited.

TIME FRAME

20–30 minutes.

MATERIALS NEEDED

Physical setting amenable to both indoor and outdoor walking, ideally near a park or public walking trail. Participants will need comfortable walking shoes and appropriate outdoor clothing.

PROCESS

1. Announce that participants will be taking a short walk outdoors and indoors to explore the ways that sensory awareness can enhance the body/mind benefits of exercise.

2. Survey the group to see how many people enjoy regular exercise or movement, and invite responders to share examples of the positive benefits they have received from exercise. Summarize these benefits in a short chalktalk.

   ● **Exercise improves body/mind health.** It restores your body to its optimum condition, so you can live actively and happily. Regular exercise can increase energy, improve cardiovascular fitness, develop greater endurance and flexibility, reduce stress, strengthen your immune system, clear your thinking (including increased creativity in problem solving), and evoke a brighter outlook on life.

   ● **Exercise heightens sensory awareness.** In the natural high of exercise you can let go of your worries and focus on the sensory pleasures of the moment: the feel of wind on your face when you ski downhill, the smell of autumn leaves when you walk in the woods, the brilliance of sunlight on the waves as you jog down the beach, the feel of the water as you swim across the pool, or the mellow sounds of music as you dance with a partner.

3. Point out the positive functions of our senses and the power of sensory awareness as you continue the chalktalk.

⬤ **Our senses act as bridges between body and mind.** You see the ocean and find yourself quieting down inside; you listen to space music and your brain starts making alpha waves; you smell crayons and are transported back to memories of your school days; you taste caffeine and your nervous system is aroused; you touch yourself gently and your wounds start to heal. The five physical senses link your external and internal experiences.

⬤ **Senses are essential for survival.** The smell of smoke awakens you from a deep sleep and propels you to get out of a burning house; the sound of a car horn blaring makes you slam on the brakes at an intersection; the sight of a stranger approaching at night alerts you to be careful and guard against assault; food tastes spoiled and you throw it away; a certain kind of touch feels bad and you back away from the person touching you. Your senses tell you when it's time to take action to protect yourself.

⬤ **Senses regulate automatic physiological responses.** When your senses communicate threat or danger, your sympathetic nervous system will become aroused so you become alert, tense, and pre-pared for action. When your senses communicate pleasure and safety, your parasympathetic nervous system produces endorphins that make you feel calm and quiet inside. Sensory input is the foundation of your ability to manage stress.

⬤ **Senses reinforce memory and learning.** Many of us learned the alphabet by singing the ABC rhyme over and over. We remember directions to a friend's house by the visual marker of a corner grocery instead of markings on a map. We learn to modify our eating habits by paying attention to the taste of foods high in sodium. Everyone knows the smell of a skunk in the backyard means *stay away*. Yoga is learned by the feel of your body in certain positions, the touch of your spine as it rests on the floor. Senses anchor memories in your body and mind.

⬤ **Senses enhance behavior change through pleasure.** We are more likely to continue doing something when it's fun. If exercise makes you feel alive and rejuvenated, you are likely to keep doing it. If massage makes you feel wonderful, you are probably going to seek out this pleasurable touch. If you can visualize yourself performing well in a new situation, you are more likely to risk change. If you enjoy the taste of a new, low-fat recipe, you might choose to cook other new foods that are healthy for you. If this new food smells good, it will be even more appealing.

4. Invite participants to experience the sensual pleasures of a walk outdoors, focusing on external sensory experiences, and then indoors, focusing on internal sensory experiences. Ask participants to perform a quick subjective measure of their current body/mind state before going on the walk.

   ➤ Close your eyes, take a deep breath, and allow yourself to become quiet. Use your sensory awareness to explore your *current* feeling of body/mind health. Consider your physical state, your energy level, your mood, and your mental outlook.

      ➢ On a scale of 0-10, with *0* meaning *feeling so **bad** you want to go home and go to bed,* and *10* meaning you *feel so **good** you want to sing and dance,* how well do you feel?

      ➢ Pick a number representing your current feeling, and remember it.

5. When participants have completed their subjective pre-walk health rating, offer guidelines for the outdoor walk.

   ☞ *Give suggestions on where to walk, making sure everyone understands directions so nobody gets lost.*

   ➤ If you brought walking shoes with you, go ahead and put them on now.

   ➤ Take a 10-minute walk outdoors, focusing on the pleasures of your five physical senses.

      ➢ Concentrate on the sights, sounds, smells, tastes, and touches of your surroundings. Notice the smell of air, the feel of the elements, the textures beneath your feet, the views along your route, the taste on your lips, the ever-changing sounds in the background or foreground.

      ➢ If you notice your attention wandering away from your current sensory experience, gently bring your attention back to the present moment and the data you are receiving from your five senses.

   ➤ After 10 minutes, return to the building and continue to walk around inside this room until all have returned.

6. When all participants have returned, give instructions for the indoor walk.

   ➤ Spend the next 5 minutes walking indoors.

➤ During your indoor walk, turn your attention inwards and focus on your internal sensory experiences.

> ☞ *Explain options of walking in the building (eg, meeting room, skywalks, hallways, etc).*

➤ Try to experience different parts of your body, from head to foot, from the inside out, as you walk. How does the top of your head feel? Your forehead? Eyes? Cheeks? Mouth? Jaw? Teeth? Tongue? Neck? Shoulders? Spine? And so on all throughout your body, down to the feel of your toes as you walk across the floor.

➤ If your attention starts to wander, gently pull your focus back to the sensory experience of your body as you walk, without judging yourself.

➤ After 5 minutes, return to this space and your place.

7. When all have returned, ask participants to rate their current body/mind health. Invite them to pair up and share a bit about their external and internal sensory experiences.

➤ Close your eyes, focus your attention inward, and notice your current energy, mood, and outlook.

> Rate your current level of body/mind health on a scale of 0–10, with *0* meaning you *feel so **bad** you want to go home,* and *10* meaning you *feel so **good** you want to sing and dance.*

8. Invite participants to share examples of how the walks affected their body/mind health scores, and then ask participants to share surprises and discoveries from their walks.

9. Summarize participants' responses in a final chalktalk about the power of sensory awareness and the importance of staying connected to our sensory experiences.

● **The power of awareness is one of your most precious allies** in the journey toward health. Many of us live in a state of chronic distraction. We get so busy or tense that we miss vital signs and signals from our senses: the sore muscles that tell us to slow down; the afternoon fatigue that tells us to take a break, get some fresh air; the pain in our chest that tells us to see a doctor. Listening to your senses can save your life.

● **Awareness is essential for joyful living.** Simple sensory pleasures await us when we stop deferring happiness, and decide to enjoy what is already here, in the present moment. When you take time to smell the flowers, dig in the earth with your hands to plant a garden, watch the chickadees on your birdfeeder, taste the rain on your tongue, and listen to the leaves rustle in the wind, you are rewarded with moments of wonder, peace, and delight.

- **Enjoy sensual walks everyday.**When you walk from your car or bus to your office, get sensual. Notice the color of the sky, the sounds of your feet on the pavement, the feel of your muscles moving on your hips. Use your next coffee break to take a sensual stroll outdoors, even if it is just a 5-minute jaunt down the block. Enjoy the feel of inhaling fresh air, and the relief of blowing away stale, gray air. Have fun, and enjoy your senses!

FOR ONGOING GROUPS

- Incorporate short, sensory experiences into your group: a 5-minute body-scan for tension, a 3-minute meditation, a 10-minute sensual walk, etc.

- Plan a special mini-session focused on each of the five senses: touch, taste, smell, sight, and sound. Use the creativity of the group to make up interesting, fun exercises.

This exercise was contributed by Mary O'Brien Sippel.

23 PAST CONNECTIONS

This quiet, reflective process uses journaling methods to explore connections between past events and current food and body issues.

GOALS

To increase awareness of the relationship between life events and the use of food.

To explore the effects of personal history on body image.

To develop a broad perspective of personal struggles with food and body issues.

GROUP SIZE

Unlimited.

TIME FRAME

40–50 minutes.

MATERIALS NEEDED

Blank paper or journals; **Focusing** script; **Past Connections** worksheets.

PROCESS

1. Set the stage for this reflection process by expanding the concept of time.

   ● **Time is the period when something occurs.** An event happens, a process begins, lasts a moment or a decade, and then ends. It is the way we measure the movement of our lives. You might say, *It was a hard time in my life,* when you refer to your days as a fat teenager, or the years of an unhappy marriage. Or you might say, *Those were happy times,* when you recall your college years, the discovery of your identity, or the years when your children were toddlers.

   ● **Time is elastic.** The here and now is not just the present moment. The *now* stretches back as far as it needs to go to include whatever portion of the past that is still active in the present. The *now* includes all aspects of the past that are a meaningful part of our present experience. The *now* also includes our images of the future that affect the present: plans, hopes, worries, and dreams.

● **There are two kinds of time:** chronological time and qualitative time. *Chronological time* refers to the order in which events occur. We assign dates or numbers to mark events in time. *Qualitative time* is the *subjective* perception of objective events in terms of the meaning and value they have for you. When we say "I remember it like it was yesterday," we are saying that this event still holds power for the present.

2. Distribute blank paper (or journals) for recording responses. Announce that participants will be using meditation and journaling to explore both *chronological* and *qualitative* events that are a part of their current food and body dilemma.

   ➤ Identify the period of your life in which you have been *struggling with food and body issues.*

   ➤ As you tune in to this period of your life, focus on the *general feeling* of your life instead of thinking about it or analyzing the details.

      ➤ Don't judge your feelings, just notice them. Don't try to direct your feelings, just be aware of them.

      ➤ You may see images, think of metaphors, hear music, feel strong emotions during this experience. Whatever happens will be unique to you and exactly right for you.

      ➤ Trust yourself and your perceptions. Do not censor them unless they are too disturbing to you.

   ➤ If you start to feel distressed or scared, open your eyes.

3. Read the **Focusing** script, pausing as indicated for images to form.

4. When most participants have returned their attention to the room, encourage them to record their images while they are fresh.

   ➤ On your blank sheet of paper (or journal) write or draw the words, feelings, sounds, or images that came to you as you reflected on your struggles with food and body image.

   ☞ *Allow 4–5 minutes for individual writing and drawing.*

5. After 5 minutes, pass out **Past Connections** worksheets and explain the steps for further reflection.

   ➤ In the left column, labeled **Life Events,** briefly list (one or two word descriptions) all of the significant life events that have been or are a part of this period of your struggle with food and body. Feel free to add whatever events pop into your mind.

☞ *Prime the pump with examples for several categories of life events.*

Physical: illness, accidents, puberty, menopause, body size, athletic achievement, abuse.

Mental: scholastic ability, artistic achievement, negative thoughts about body, put downs by family.

Social: family moving, parents' divorce, loss of friends, new job.

Emotional: mother's depression, brother's rage, punishment for sharing feelings.

Spiritual: religious experiences, death of friend.

Cultural: Twiggy as role model, stereotyping of women, fatism, racism.

➤ Estimate the chronological order of these events by writing the date or year by the event.

➤ If you are uncertain of the date, make a guess based on your age when the event occurred. If you wish, you can check out the accuracy later by talking with family members, reviewing school records, etc.

6. When most participants have finished listing life events (about 5 minutes), give additional instructions for exploring food and body connections to these events.

➤ In the right column labeled **Food and Body Connections,** write any food or body issue that surfaced, or problems that developed, at the time of each event you listed.

☞ *Give examples appropriate to your audience.*
Did you start overeating at the time of your father's affair?
Did you start to hate your body in the first grade when kids teased you for being fat?
Did you start dieting when you entered puberty and your breasts developed?
Did you gain 50 pounds after an assault?
Did you start bingeing and purging to meet weight requirements for gymnastics or wrestling?

➤ Search for connections in your mind. Don't worry about factual accuracy, since these are your subjective perceptions about the meaning of these events in your life.

☞ *Allow about 5 minutes for participants to explore food and body connections.*

7. Announce that participants will have the opportunity to share their story with one other person. Give instructions for small group discussion.

> Pair up with someone you do not know well.

>> Decide who will be *Past* and who will be *Present.*

>> *Presents* go first. Share whatever you want about your food and body history or story.

>> *Pasts* provide confidentiality, respect, acceptance, and attentive listening.

After 3 minutes, I will give the signal to switch roles.

☞ *Announce when 3 minutes are up and it's time to switch partners.*

> *Pasts* tell your stories while *Presents* listen and keep confidentiality.

8. After 6 minutes, interrupt the pairs and ask participants to rejoin the large group. Encourage participants to continue sharing their discoveries later with selected close friends, family, support group, therapist, or other trustworthy people in their lives.

9. Conclude by encouraging participants to try journaling as a way of continuing to search for connections between life events, their use of food, and body attitudes.

● **Journaling can deepen and broaden your perspective.** Consider keeping a journal focused on this period in your life. Fill in the blanks, search for connections between life changes, stress, and body image. Your awareness of the multiple forces affecting your relationship with food and your body may help you to appreciate yourself and strengthen your ability to cope and care for yourself during stressful times.

● **Journals reveal patterns over time.** Their purpose is not to store evidence of your failures, but to preserve information about what has meaning for you. Never judge what you write. Make your journal a safe home for your deepest thoughts and feelings.

FOR ONGOING GROUPS

■ This exercise can be done in the early stages of group process, as long as basic trust, confidentiality, and safety issues are established. Encourage sharing of personal examples with the whole group in *Step 8.*

■ Use the **Past Connections** worksheet for homework between sessions.

■ Select one past event from each participant's life to focus on in the group. Work on the feelings associated with this event and challenge negative thoughts and beliefs that might underscore the individual's negative feelings.

This exercise was contributed by Rebecca Ruggles Radcliffe, author of **Enlightened Eating: Understanding and Changing Your Relationship with Food** *Minneapolis: EASE, 1996).*

FOCUSING Script

Close your eyes . . . relax quietly . . .
and turn your attention inward . . .
Focus on the movement of your life . . .
and the struggles you may have had with food . . .
or your body.

☞ *Pause 10 seconds.*

Ask yourself, where am I now in my life . . .
in my relationship with food and my body?

☞ *Pause 10 seconds.*

Allow the answer to shape itself in general terms
behind your conscious mind . . .
Let yourself inwardly feel the movement of your life
as it has been taking shape during this period of time.

☞ *Pause 20 seconds.*

As you continue to relax . . .
and reflect on this period of your life . . .
the boundaries and characteristics of this time
may start to take shape for you . . .
What events mark it off? . . .
How far back does it reach? . . .
What are the main characteristics of this period?

☞ *Pause 20 seconds.*

Sit quietly . . . and feel the inner movement
of your experience without judgement . . .
Let the quality of your experience during this time express itself to you . . .
Perhaps it will come in the form of an image . . . a metaphor . . .
a simile . . . a word . . . phrase . . . or sound that represents your reality.

☞ *Pause 20 seconds.*

Allow your images, thoughts, and feelings to take shape in your mind . . .
Simply notice what you are seeing, hearing, or feeling.

☞ *Pause 20 seconds.*

When you have these images, thoughts, or feelings focused in your mind,
prepare to return to your surroundings . . .
Slowly open your eyes . . .
and bring this awareness with you back to the present moment.

PAST CONNECTIONS

Life Events   **Food & Body Connections**

_____   _____

_____   _____

_____   _____

_____   _____

_____   _____

_____   _____

_____   _____

_____   _____

_____   _____

_____   _____

_____   _____

_____   _____

_____   _____

_____   _____

_____   _____

_____   _____

_____   _____

_____   _____

_____   _____

_____   _____

_____   _____

_____   _____

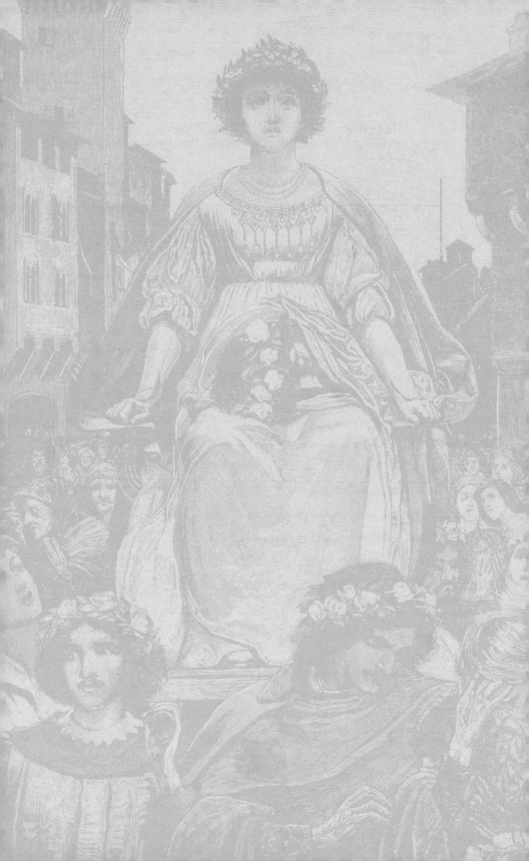

FOCUS ON
ATTITUDES:
CULTURAL & PERSONAL

These exercises challenge participants to look at their own attitudes about food and eating, body size, appearance, dieting, beauty, fat people, and overall definitions of health, from both a personal and a cultural perspective. Processes are designed to stimulate thinking, raise consciousness, and stretch participants' (and trainers') attitudes from traditional views of weight and body size to new attitudes that are based on increased respect for diversity, including body size.

24 WHAT'S MY FOCUS? page 124
This behavior assessment can be used by anyone who wants to embrace health and well-being instead of dieting and weight conflicts. (25–30 min.)

25 FAT ATTITUDES page 131
Participants examine their attitudes toward fat people, then discuss ways to build empathy and support for large people in our society. (45–60 min.)

26 MYTHS AND REALITIES page 136
Participants explore eight common myths related to health, weight, and dieting, and then explore ways to make new beliefs a reality in their lives. (45–60 min.)

27 BEAUTY CHANT page 144
This Navajo chant from the *Blessing Way* ceremony is a simple, yet powerful dance of affirmation and support for participants. (15–20 min.)

28 FAT CHANCE page 148
Participants work in small groups to create outrageous responses to situations that challenge a size-accepting lifestyle. (15–20 min.)

29 WHO SAYS SO? page 153
In this lively Greek chorus, participants shout down cultural stereotypes and challenge negative body beliefs. (10–20 min.)

24 WHAT'S MY FOCUS?

This behavior assessment can be used by anyone who wants to embrace health and well-being instead of diet and weight conflicts.

GOALS

To explore personal focus, attitudes, and behavior related to physical appearance and human value.

To set specific goals for healthier attitudes toward self and others.

GROUP SIZE

Unlimited.

TIME FRAME

25–30 minutes.

MATERIALS NEEDED

What's My Focus? questionnaires.

PROCESS

1. Give a brief chalktalk about how life focus affects personal health and well-being, and shapes cultural norms and values about size, appearance, and human worth.

   ● **We are what we focus on.** Our preoccupations tell a lot about ourselves: our beliefs, values, and attitudes. If you are preoccupied with making money, and most of your time and energy is devoted to money-making ventures, you are choosing a focus on material wealth. If you do a lot of daydreaming, you may be choosing to dwell in the past or future instead of your present reality. If your primary life goal is to lose weight, you may be choosing to forgo pleasures or activities you could enjoy at your current weight.

   ● **Focus can be healthy or unhealthy.** It's healthy to focus on your diet and the condition of your body when this vigilance keeps you motivated to pay attention to your overall health and zest for life. It's not healthy to get so focused on food or your body that the preoccupation consumes most of your time and attention, leaving little energy for other projects or people you care about.

   ● **Negative focus can be changed to positive focus.** If you focus on the negative, you are more likely to feel depressed, anxious, or discouraged. Shifting to a positive focus will empower you to move on with your life and move ahead with your goals. For example, if you have been negatively focused on your dress size, this will slow you down and make you feel bad. If you shift your focus to becoming more physically fit or flexible, you'll be better able to enjoy your body, regardless of your dress size.

2. Invite participants to examine their own focus on body size, shape, and appearance by completing a questionnaire developed by Susan Kano, author of *Making Peace With Food*. Hand out **What's My Focus?** questionnaires and explain how to complete them.

> For each item on the questionnaire, circle the letter that represents how often you do that behavior.

>> **N** = Never, **R** = Rarely, **O** = Occasionally, **F** = Frequently, **D** = Daily.

>> *Someone* includes anyone—from a stranger to a friend or family member, anyone—except yourself.

3. After most people have completed the questionnaire, ask for insights.

> Look over the questions in **Column 1** on the first page of your worksheet. What do you notice?

☞ *Solicit ideas. Emphasize that these are **unhelpful** behaviors and attitudes.*

> Look at the questions in **Column 2**. What do you notice?

☞ *Solicit ideas. Point out that these are **helpful** behaviors and attitudes.*

4. Give a brief chalktalk about the *unhelpful* and *helpful* behaviors and attitudes described in **Columns 1** and **2**.

● **Focus on size and appearance is not always helpful.** In fact, attention to physical qualities may be hurtful, since it reinforces cultural beliefs that appearance is more important than competence, that thinness is better than fatness, and that people who do not fit cultural ideals for appearance or body size should be singled out or devalued in some way. Taken to an extreme, a focus on size and appearance can drive some people to do things that are unhealthy for them—such as skipping meals to lose weight.

● **Focus on positive qualities is helpful.** Accentuating the positive will build positive, loving relationships with people in your family, workplace, and community. It will reduce incidents of size discrimination and increase experiences that are affirming and inclusive for people of all sizes. And it will put the focus on what counts: people, not pounds.

5. Invite participants to explore their personal need for changing from an *unhelpful* focus to a *more helpful* one.

> ➤ Look over your responses in **Column 1** of your worksheet. Consider setting a personal goal to change unhelpful behaviors and attitudes.

> ➤ Select at least three focus items that you want to change. For each item, write a personal goal for changing from an *unhelpful* to a *helpful* focus. Use the space below the item to write your goal.

> ☞ *Ask participants to give examples of how to change some of the items. For example, if your pattern has been to encourage dieting, you could remind yourself and others that what is most important is how you are feeling, physically and emotionally.*

6. Invite participants to explore *underutilized helpful* focuses.

> ➤ Look at your answers for the items in **Column 2** on your worksheet. All of these actions can be helpful. For each item where you circled **N** or **R** (for Never or Rarely), consider setting personal goals to increase that behavior.

> ➤ Identify at least three *helpful* behaviors that you want to *increase,* and identify personal goals for how to do this. Use the space below the selected items to write your goal.

7. Invite participants to look more closely at the items in **Column 3**, providing guidelines for transforming these *typically unhelpful* cultural attitudes into a *more helpful* focus. Encourage participants to make note of any appealing strategies for change.

> ● **Appearance.** Talking about appearance is natural, but it is excessive in our culture. Focus on appearance objectifies people (especially women) and encourages the development of exaggerated concern about body weight and size. We need to realize (and teach others) that appearance is less important than health, happiness, and character.

> ● **Slenderness.** Appreciating the physical beauty of slender people is fine, provided that you do not promote the idea that slenderness is a prerequisite for beauty. Appreciate the beauty of fat and pudgy people just as often as skinny ones. Remember to minimize all appearance-oriented comments.

> ● **Exercise.** Regular exercise is a great way to promote good health and well-being, but extreme exercising for weight control is unhealthy. Talk about exercise as a personal choice for having fun and feeling good, instead of a prescription for losing body fat or becoming a better (more disciplined) person.

- **Weight.** Discussions about weight can be positive if they refute popular myths or appreciate how helpful and healthy it has been for someone to stop dieting and maintain a comfortable, stable weight. It is harmful to talk about weight when it provokes shame or encourages unhealthy behavior and unrealistic goals.

- **Calories.** It can be helpful to expose nutritional myths, but discussions about the calorie content of food are usually unnecessary, unhelpful, and often harmful. Only *dieters* worry and talk about calories. Don't encourage others to continue in a *dieter* mentality.

- **Diets.** Talking about your hunger is fine, but whenever you focus on meager eating as a personal triumph, need, or goal, you promote the destructive culture of dieting.

- **Perfectionism.** In general, perfection is an unrealistic and destructive goal. Many (but not all) people who struggle with food issues or fragile self-esteem are trapped in striving for perfection. Instead of reinforcing this cycle, encourage all people to appreciate themselves and their accomplishments however *imperfect* they may be.

- **Conformity.** If everyone constantly tried to conform to current societal norms and expectations about body weight and appearance, the epidemic of eating disorders would be of even larger proportions. Support the people around you as they tune in to their own values and make decisions based on inner integrity rather than outward conformity.

- **Criticism.** When you recognize a problem and imagine a possible solution feel free to offer it. However, stress your suggestion rather than your criticism; focus on choices or behaviors rather than the person. Be cautious in your judgments and strategy with faultfinding. Be sure to balance criticism with sincere, positive statements so the person feels appreciated.

8. Ask participants to reflect further on changes they want to make.

   ➤ Summarize your resolutions for change under the **Changing My Focus Resolutions Column** on page 2 of your worksheet.

      ➤ Note *unhelpful* behaviors you want to *decrease*.

9. After 2–5 minutes, ask participants to write a plan for implementing these changes in focus.

   ➤ Look over your list of resolutions for change. Write a final statement for what you will do **Today** and **This week** to change your focus.

      ➤ Note *helpful* behaviors you want to *continue* or *increase*.

10. Invite participants to share their focus-changing goals with another participant.

> Pair up with another group member whom you do not know well.

> Decide who will be **Health** and who will be **Wellness**.

> **Health** goes first. Share whatever you want about your goals for changing your focus, while **Wellness** listens.

> After 2 minutes, reverse roles so **Wellness** can talk about your goals while **Health** listens.

11. After 4 minutes, solicit examples and conclude with a peptalk about implementing change.

● **Work on moment-to-moment changes.** When you catch yourself making destructive comments, admit your slips but don't be hard on yourself. It takes a lot of time and practice to change habits and attitudes you've formed over many years.

● **Review your goals regularly.** For the first two weeks, review your goals twice daily; for the third week, review them every other day; for the fourth through the eighth weeks, review them once a week. This is especially important if you live with someone who is pre-occupied with diet and weight. The two of you may have developed some destructive patterns that often go unnoticed. When you review your goals, you will soon see errors and know how to correct them.

● **Continue to challenge destructive cultural messages.** Even after you have changed your own focus, you will continue to be confronted by the diet and weight focus in our culture. Periodically reviewing your goals may help counteract all the insidious advertisements, conversations, etc. By speaking out, you'll help many people who are affected by these same negative influences.

FOR ONGOING GROUPS

■ Ideal for an introduction and orientation process done in the early stages of a group.

■ Have participants retake the **What's My Focus?** questionnaire after 2–3 months of work on these issues.

*This exercise was contributed by Susan Kano, author of **Making Peace with Food** (New York: HarperCollins, 1989).*

> **8** – Imagine a figure 8 on the ground around your feet. Trace the 8 with your knees, your hips, and your shoulders, stretching as far as you can.

> **9** – Tap your seat with one hand and then the other as you say: *1–2–3–4–5–6–7–8–9: Moving makes my body feel so fine.* Repeat a second time.

3. Ask participants to pair up with a neighbor and stand facing each other for the final sequence.

   > Decide who is **Body** and who is **Count.**

   >> **Count** starts. Indicate your phone number to your partner by making the movements that go with each digit.

   >> **Body** try to figure out your partner's number by the actions.

   > Switch roles.

4. Reconvene the group and ask if anyone correctly guessed the phone number of their partner. Ask any pair who guessed correctly to stand up and take a bow, while other participants give them a standing ovation.

FOR ONGOING GROUPS

■ Make playful, fun movement a routine part of your group activity.

■ Let participants create new movement energizers, using music, spontaneous dance, or other methods dreamed up by individuals.

This exercise was contributed by Martha Belknap.

32 FANS OF MOZART

In this refreshing upper body dance routine, participants cool off while paddling down a river to a fantasy destination.

GOALS

To make a positive connection between exercise, music, and imagery.

TIME FRAME

5–10 minutes.

MATERIALS NEEDED

CD or cassette player; CD or audiotape of lively Mozart music; two paper plates for each participant; **Fans of Mozart** script.

PROCESS

☞ *Be sure to practice this routine a few times before springing it on a group.*

1. Introduce the concept of Chair Dancing® as a fun way to exercise without leaving your chair.

2. Hand out two paper plates to each participant, ask them to sit up straight in their chairs, start the music, and read the **Fans of Mozart** script, demonstrating the movements as you go.

   ☞ *To involve the lower body, add heel bounces or walking in place while seated. This breaks the myth that Chair Dancing® is only arm movements!*

*This exercise was contributed by Jodi Stolove, creator of **Chair Dancing®, A New Concept in Aerobic Fitness**. 10- and 45-minute videotapes ($19.95) and an audiocassette ($9.95) of similar routines are available from Chair Dancing® International (800-551-4FUN).*

FANS OF MOZART Script*

Put one plate in each hand. The plates are your fans.
Fan yourself with both hands . . . enjoy it . . . You've worked hard for it.
Fan yourself some more, it feels good.
Fan out to your side, fan your neighbor . . .
Now fan yourself . . . now your neighbor . . .
Fan yourself . . . now your neighbor . . . Fan yourself . . . now your neighbor.

Now fan yourself and your neighbor, in and out . . .
in and out . . . in and out . . . in and out . . .
Now fan in front of yourself . . . fan your neighbor across the way . . .
air-condition the whole room . . . up and around.
Fan behind yourself . . . fan the part you've been sitting on . . . it feels good.

Put your plates together inside each other . . .
and hold them together with both hands.
They're your paddles now . . . and you're in a canoe.
Reach forward and to the right with your plates to paddle.
Stroke down and back propelling your canoe forward.
Now take a stroke on the left side . . . forward . . . down . . . back . . .

Keep paddling, alternating sides.
Where will you go? . . . What water are we in?
Paddle on the right . . . paddle on the left . . .
Is it a beautiful stream, or river, or rapids?
Paddle on the right for two strokes . . . paddle on the left for two strokes . . .
Now paddle one each side, right and left . . . right and left

Now separate your plates and hold one on each side again . . .
Fan yourself . . . fan your neighbor . . . Fan yourself . . . fan your neighbor . . .
Fan yourself . . . fan your neighbor . . . Fan yourself . . . fan your neighbor . . .

Now fan yourself and your neighbor . . . fan in and out . . . in and out . . .
Fan in front of yourself . . . fan your neighbor across the way . . .
air-condition the whole room, up and down.
Fan behind yourself . . . fan where you've been sitting . . . it feels good.

Put your plates together again, they're your paddles again.
Stroke on the right . . . stroke on your left . . .
Shall we paddle to Hawaii, Tahiti, Venice, or the Riviera?
Paddle on your right . . . paddle on your left . . .
Paddle on your right for two . . . and your left for two . . .
on your right . . . and your left.
Paddle one on each side, we're almost there . . . Let's go!
Keep paddling . . . I see land . . . We'll get there if you keep paddling . . .
We've arrived!! Let's go ashore!

* Script from Jodi Stolove, creator of **Chair Dancing**®.

33 FIGHT SONG

Participants create unique cheers challenging size discrimination and promoting size acceptance.

GOALS

To build camaraderie and support for non-dieting, size-accepting behaviors and attitudes.

GROUP SIZE

Unlimited. Works best with several small groups of 4–6 people.

TIME FRAME

10–15 minutes.

MATERIALS NEEDED

Fight Song examples; blank paper.

PROCESS

1. Ask participants to rejoin small groups from a previous exercise or, if you wish, form new small groups of 4–6 people. Give each group several sheets of blank paper.

2. When groups are settled, explain that each team will be creating a fight song or cheer that advocates an end to size discrimination, dieting, or negative body attitudes.

    ☞ *Give several examples from the samples on p. 165 or make up your own.*

    ➤ You have 5 minutes to pick a theme, create your cheer, and rehearse it before performing it for the group.

    ➢ Feel free to copy the style or rhythm of one of the sample cheers or model your creation after a cheer from your school days.

3. After 5 minutes, invite each group to stand up and perform its cheer.

This exercise was contributed by Sally Strosahl who learned the cheers at a NAAFA Convention.

FOR ONGOING GROUPS

■ This is a fun, nonthreatening way for participants to play together while actively challenging negative beliefs about weight and body size.

■ Best used as a follow-up to discussions about the negative effects of yo-yo dieting and fat-ism in our culture.

FIGHT SONG examples

Fat and happy
Fat and proud
All together
Sing it loud.

Hit 'em high
Hit 'em low
The diet deception's got to go.

Regulate!
Legislate!
Do it now, it's not too late!

One, two, three
What's it gonna be?
Four, five, six
Give up your bag of tricks
Seven, eight, nine
Dieting's a waste of time.

One, two, three, four
Respect is what we're fighting for
Five, six, seven, eight
Accept yourself at any weight.

34 SNACK CAFETERIA

Participants turn snack-time into an opportunity for learning, using a mini-cafeteria to explore the kinesthetic, visual, and cognitive aspects of informed food choices.

GOALS

To connect internal hunger cues with visual and cognitive aspects of choosing food.

To practice making good decisions about food while enjoying a nourishing break.

TIME FRAME

20 minutes.

MATERIALS NEEDED

Variety of serving-size snack foods, chosen in advance by the trainer, laid out on a long table, labeled by serving sizes with whatever nutritional information the trainer wants to emphasize (eg, calories, fat, carbohydrates, protein, vitamins, calcium, salt, sugar, etc) or according to a food exchange program of the trainer's choice. There should be sufficient portions so participants can choose more than one serving. Include fruit, cheese, pretzels, chips, nuts, cookies, crackers, candy, yogurt, muffins, juice, milk, coffee.

Menus prepared in advance by the trainer, listing all foods and beverages in the cafeteria; **Nutrition Values** handout prepared in advance, summarizing nutritional content (eg, calories, fat grams, mg of sodium, vitamins, food exchange, etc) of all foods and beverages on the **Menus; Nutrition Basics** handout, prepared by the trainer, outlining basic nutritional information you want to highlight.

PROCESS

☞ *Remind chronic dieters or overeaters who are in the process of legalizing food or otherwise trying to break free from obsessive patterns in their eating to use this experience as an opportunity for exercising freedom of choice and tuning in to their hungers.*

1. Start by guiding participants in a short relaxation exercise to tune in to hunger.

   ➤ Take a minute to close your eyes and relax.

➤ Allow yourself to become quiet, let your breathing become slow and deep, breathing in through your nose, and out through your mouth.

➤ Tune in to your current level of hunger, down in your belly. Listen for hunger sensations, and decide how hungry you are using a hunger scale, with 0 for famished and 10 for so full you can't move.

➤ Rate your hunger level in your mind, then slowly open your eyes.

2. Hand out **Menus** to all participants, and explain that all foods and beverages on the **Menu** are available in the snack cafeteria. Invite participants to think about what they want to eat during this snack.

➤ Keeping in mind your current hunger level, look over the menu and decide what foods and/or beverages you want for your snack.

➤ For each choice, be sure to estimate the number of servings that will satisfy your current hunger and thirst.

➤ When you have decided what you want, go ahead and walk through the snack cafeteria line, reading the nutritional information posted by each food and beverage item as you make your selections.

➤ Feel free to add or skip food items, or change portion sizes as you go through the cafeteria line.

➤ Help yourself to whatever you imagine will satisfy your hunger and thirst.

➤ Find a comfortable space to enjoy your snack, eating as much as you'd like without criticizing or judging your food choices.

3. When most people have finished their snack, distribute **Nutrition Values** for the menu items, and ask participants to use this as a guide for evaluating the snack just consumed.

➤ Record the serving sizes of all your snacks, using the **Nutrition Values** handout to determine the nutritional content of your snack.

➤ Then, for each nutritional value (eg, calories, grams of fat, food exchange, mg of sodium, vitamins, etc) calculate the total for your snack and record it on your **Menu.**

4. Give everyone a **Nutrition Basics** handout. Suggest that they review it and use it as a resource for future reflection about their snack choices.

5. Invite participants to share what they learned in the exercise.

➤ Pair up with a neighbor and talk about your insights and observations about hunger level, selecting snacks, and nutritional values.

➤ Take about 2 minutes each.

6. Solicit observations from the group, incorporating responses into a closing reminder about the importance of integrating kinesthetic, visual, and cognitive information into eating choices.

● **Develop an integrated approach to eating.** Use your body to identify hunger levels before you eat. Look at the size of each portion, and compare it with abstract data about nutritional values of that particular food and portion size. Use your mind to integrate knowledge about nutrition with visual cues of what serving sizes *look like* on your plate. Balance this cognitive and visual knowledge with your internal hunger. Seek a balance between all of these dimensions so no one aspect of eating dominates your choices.

FOR ONGOING GROUPS

■ Use the **Snack Cafeteria** routinely as an opportunity to practice making integrated, healthy food choices. Vary the foods and nutritional focus each time. If possible, plan a complete *mealtime cafeteria* so a wider variety of foods can be integrated.

■ Have participants make up other games using the cafeteria process to make learning about nutrition fun and practical.

35 MINDFUL EATING EXPERIENCE

When participants eat with full awareness, eating becomes a satisfying, sensory experience that is both relaxing and nourishing.

GOALS

To learn a relaxing, pleasurable style of eating.

To enjoy nourishing food.

GROUP SIZE

Unlimited.

TIME FRAME

5–15 minutes.

MATERIALS NEEDED

Fresh, juicy oranges for all participants, cut into 1/8 sections (with skins) immediately before serving; paper towels. Optional: include a variety of other foods, such as raisins, peanuts, baked tortilla chips, grapes, or Hershey's Kisses.

PROCESS

1. Give a short chalktalk explaining the concept and skill of mindfulness.

   ● **Mindfulness is a relaxation skill.** When you are mindful, you focus all of your attention on what you are doing or experiencing at the present moment. You concentrate completely, so that all other distractions are blocked out or ignored. This helps you relax and enjoy the sensory pleasures of the moment: the sights, sounds, smells, touches, and tastes of your world.

   ● **Mindfulness is a natural skill.** Watch a baby examine a new object, and you will see mindfulness in its purest form. If you enjoy artistic, creative pursuits like painting, sculpting, pottery, dance, music, and other arts, you have probably enjoyed the deeply restorative, satisfying effects of this kind of attentiveness. Sewing on a button, washing the dishes, skiing down a snowy hill, listening to the wind rustle autumn leaves, and many other simple, sensory experiences can be approached from a mindful state of being.

2. Announce that participants will have the opportunity to refresh mentally and physically, using a mindful eating experience. Give each partici-

pant an orange section and a paper towel with a reminder to wait for instruction before eating. Explain that you will be guiding the group through several steps of a relaxed eating process.

> ☞ *Don't rush. Allow plenty of time for participants to savor each step of this process. This step should take at least 5 minutes and could be stretched to 10 or more.*

➤ Make yourself as comfortable as possible.

➤ Take a deep breath, way down into your abdomen, causing your tummy to rise slowly as you fill yourself with air.

➤ Slowly exhale through your mouth, letting your stomach fall slowly as you empty yourself of air and releasing tension as you blow quietly outward.

➤ Take another deep breath, again filling yourself with air, and slowly release it with a deep, relaxing breath, blowing away tension as you exhale.

➤ As you continue to breathe slowly and deeply, focus your attention on your orange section.

  ➤ Pick up the piece of orange and hold it in your hand. Close your eyes and explore its shape and texture with your hands.

  ➤ Still keeping your eyes closed, lift the orange up to your face and gently touch it to your cheek. Notice how it feels on your face— and in your hand.

➤ Now open your eyes and look at the section of orange more closely. Look again at its shape, color, texture. What is it like?

➤ Now peel the skin from your orange section. Pay attention to the feeling of its skin as you pull it away from the orange. Notice the looks of the fruit inside.

  ➤ Take a piece of the skin and put it up to your nose and smell it, breathing in deeply.

➤ When you have your section completely peeled, discard the skin and focus on the fruit.

  ➤ Pick the orange up and smell it again.

  ➤ Now hold your orange section up to the light. What does it look like?

➤ Now take a small bite of your orange section and hold it in your mouth a few seconds, without biting down. Close your eyes and explore the feeling, texture, taste, and smell of it in your mouth.

➤ Now go ahead and bite down fully, noticing the changing sensations you experience as your teeth crush the fruit.

    ➤ Chew slowly, savoring each morsel as you move it around in your mouth.

    ➤ Then swallow it.

➤ Continue to eat as much as you want of the rest of your orange. Concentrate on the pleasure of eating, allowing yourself to relax and sink into the experience as much as possible.

3. If you want, introduce other small food (eg, raisins, Hershey's Kisses, or taco chips) and guide participants through the mindful eating process for each food.

4. Invite participants to share their reactions to these eating experiences, and then summarize the benefits of mindful eating in a short chalktalk.

    ● **Mindful eating helps prevent overeating.** When you are relaxed and attentive to your sensory experiences in the present moment, you are more attuned to your body, your hunger, and satiety levels. You are more likely to know what satisfies you—and when you have had enough. By slowing down the process of eating, you allow your brain the 20-minute time period it needs to recognize *fullness,* and send the signal *enough* back to you.

FOR ONGOING GROUPS

▪ Work on this skill and pleasure in group, trying a variety of foods or even a meal that participants plan and eat together.

▪ Encourage participants to practice mindful eating at home, and develop practical strategies for making their eating experiences as relaxing as possible. (Music, tablecloth, ground rules about table conversations and manners at mealtime such as no telephone calls, no unpleasant topics, no reading or watching TV while eating, etc).

This exercise was contributed by Geneen Roth, author of **When Food Is Love** *(New York: Plume/Penguin Books USA, Inc, 1991).*

36 EMPTY CALORIES

This tongue-in-cheek reading pokes fun at calorie-counting obsessions.

GOALS

To affirm the importance of exercise while finding humor in calorie counting.

TIME FRAME

5–10 minutes.

MATERIALS NEEDED

Empty Calories list.

PROCESS

1. Poll the group to see how many participants would describe their job as sedentary. Then invite people to consider amusing ways to burn calories in a sedentary job.

2. Encourage participants to burn calories by *getting a kick out of it* as you read some examples from the **Empty Calories** list.

   ☞ *These calories are mythical not actual. Remind folks that most people burn approximately 100 calories/hour while sedentary.*

3. Unless the group is extremely uptight, ask participants to get up and try some of the activities from the **Empty Calories** list. Select two or three activities that you think would be fun to try, then guide participants through a nonverbal acting-out of the chosen activities.

   ☞ *Encourage people to exaggerate the movements, letting themselves be silly for a moment.*

4. Remind participants that the true health benefits of exercise don't come from counting calories.

   ● **Regular exercise changes the body chemistry** so that you make more muscle and less fat from your food, and burn more fat more efficiently—even when you're sedentary.

   ● **Regular exercise strengthens the heart muscle**, increasing its capacity, efficiency, and endurance.

5. Invite participants to burn even more calories by *playing ball* with you and *jumping in with both feet* as you move on to the next group agenda.

EMPTY CALORIES

Activity	Calories/hour
Beating around the bush	50
Climbing the walls	175
Swallowing your pride	25
Jumping to conclusions	75
Passing the buck	25
Throwing your weight around	100-300
Bending over backwards	40
Pushing your luck	200
Making mountains from molehills	350
Tooting your own horn	25
Running around in circles	225
Eating crow	150
Wrapping it up for the day	120
Balancing the budget	450
Carrying the ball	175
Running late	80
Spinning your wheels	50
Falling all over yourself	130
Breaking the ice	45
Throwing a monkey wrench into it	75
Turning over a new leaf	30
Pulling up your stakes	90
Holding your horses	100
Turning the tables	250
Lifting yourself up by your bootstraps	100–300
Burying the hatchet	100
Hanging by a thread	275
Shooting the bull	75
Climbing the ladder of success	450
Blowing your top	300
Sticking your neck out	50
Getting your dander up	20
Playing ball	200
Stretching to the limit	175
Drawing the line	40
Leaving no stone unturned	220

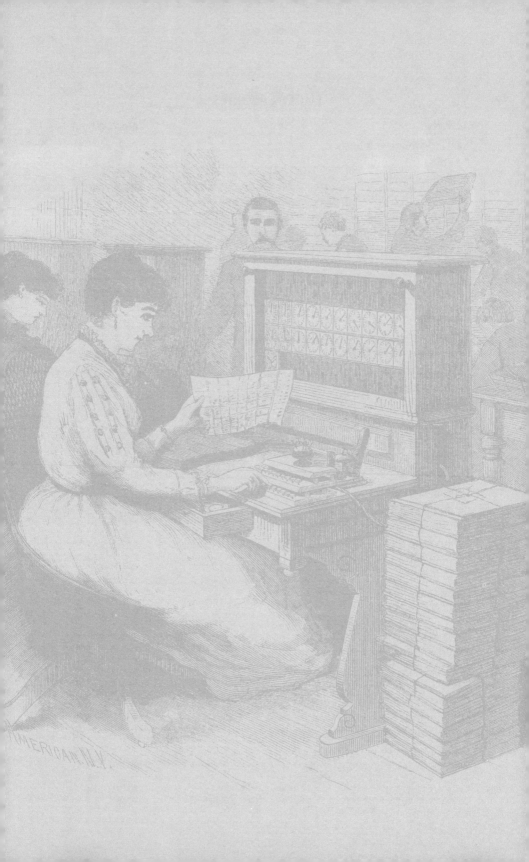

RESOURCES

This resource section provides a listing of books, magazines, newsletters, journals, organizations, videotapes, and audiocassetes related to food and body connections as well as a short, professional biography of each contributor to this book.

RESOURCE BOOKS

Ballentine, Rudolph, MD. *Diet and Nutrition: A Wholistic Approach*. Honesdale PA: Himalayan International Institute, 1984.

Bennett, William, MD, and Joel Gurin. *The Dieter's Dilemma: Eating Less and Weighing More*. New York: Basic Books, 1982.

Boston Women's Health Book Collective. *The New Our Bodies, Ourselves: A Book By and For Women*. New York: Simon and Schuster, 1992.

Brody, Jane. *Jane Brody's Nutrition Book*. New York: Bantam, 1987.

Capacchione, Lucia, and Elizabeth Johnson. *Lighten Up Journal: Making Friends With Your Body*. Santa Monica CA, 1985.

Ciliska, Donna, RN, PhD. *Beyond Dieting: Psychoeducational Interventions for Chronically Obese Women: A Non-Dieting Approach*. New York: Brunner/Mazel, 1990.

Erdman, Cheri K. *Nothing to Lose: A Guide to Sane Living in a Larger Body*. New York: HarperCollins, 1995.

Fallon, Patricia, Melanie Katzman, and Susan Wooley. *Feminist Perspectives on Eating Disorders*. New York: Guilford Press, 1994.

Hall, Lindsey, ed. *Full Lives: Women Who Have Freed Themselves from Food and Weight Obsessions*. Carlsbad CA: Gürze Books, 1993.

Hall, Lindsey, and Leigh Cohn. *Self Esteem: Tools for Recovery*. Carlsbad CA: Gürze Books, 1990.

Hirschmann, Jane R., and Carol H. Munter. *Overcoming Overeating*. New York: Fawcett Columbine, 1988.

Hirschmann, Jane R., and Carol H. Munter. *When Women Stop Hating Their Bodies: Freeing Yourself from Food and Weight Obsession*. New York: Fawcett Columbine, 1995.

Hutchinson, Marcia Germaine. *Transforming Body Image*. Freedom CA: Crossing Press, 1985.

Johnson, Carol A. *Self-Esteem Comes in All Sizes: How to Be Happy and Healthy at Your Natural Weight*. New York: Doubleday, 1995.

Kano, Susan. *Making Peace with Food*. New York: HarperCollins, 1989.

Kembel, Julie Waltz. *Winning the Weight and Wellness Game*. Tucson AZ: Northwest Learning Associates Inc, 1993.

Lyons, Pat, and Debora Burgard. *Great Shape: The First Fitness Guide for Large Women*. Palo Alto CA: Bull Publishing Company, 1990.

Newman, Lesléa, ed. *Eating Our Hearts Out: Personal Accounts of Women's Relationship to Food*. Freedom CA: Crossing Press, 1993.

Orbach, Susie. *Fat Is a Feminist Issue II: A Program to Conquer Compulsive Eating*. New York: Berkley Books, 1987.

Radcliffe, Rebecca Ruggles. *Enlightened Eating: Understanding and Changing Your Relationship with Food*. Minneapolis MN: EASE, 1993.

Roberts, Nancy. *Breaking All the Rules: Feeling Good and Looking Great No Matter What Your Size.* New York: Penguin Books, 1985.

Roth, Geneen. *Breaking Free from Compulsive Eating.* New York: Bobbs-Merrill, 1990.

Sandbeck, Terence J., PhD. *The Deadly Diet: Recovering from Anorexia and Bulimia.* Oakland CA: New Harbinger, 1986.

Somer, Elizabeth, MA, RD. *Food and Mood: The Complete Guide to Eating Well and Feeling Your Best.* New York: Henry Holt and Company, 1995.

Travis, John W., MD, and Sara Regina Ryan. *Wellness: Small Changes You Can Use to Make a Big Difference.* Berkeley CA: Ten Speed Press, 1991.

Waterhouse, Debra, MPH, RD. *Why Women Need Chocolate: Eat What You Crave to Look Good & Feel Great.* New York: Hyperion, 1995.

Wittenberg, Margaret M. *Good Food: The Complete Guide to Eating Well.* Freedom CA: Crossing Press, 1995.

Wolf, Naomi. *The Beauty Myth: How Images of Beauty Are Used Against Women.* New York: Doubleday, 1991.

RECOMMENDED MAGAZINES, NEWSLETTERS, AND JOURNALS

Big Beautiful Woman (BBW). 213-651-0469, 800-707-5592 for subscribers.

The Enlightened Eating Newsletter. EASE, PO Box 8032, Minneapolis MN 55408-0032. 612-825-7681.

EXTRA! Woman. PO Box 57194, Sherman Oaks CA 91413. 818-997-8404.

Fat! So? PO Box 423464, San Fransisco CA 94142-3464.

Food for Thought. c/o Largesse, 74 Woolsey St, PO Box 9404, New Haven CT 06534-0404. 203-787-1624 (fax and phone).

Healthy Weight Journal. Healthy Living Institute, 402 S 14th St, Hettinger ND 58639. 701-567-2646.

On a Positive Note. PO Box 17223, Glendale WI 53217.

The Overcoming Overeating Newsletter. The National Center for Overcoming Overeating, 315 W 86th St, Suite 17B, New York NY 10024. 800-299-0577.

Radiance: the Magazine for Large Women. PO Box 30246, Oakland CA 94604. 510-482-0680 (fax and phone).

RELATED ORGANIZATIONS

ABUNDIA: Programs for the Promotion of Body-Size Acceptance and Self-Esteem. PO Box 252, Downers Grove IL 60515. 708-897-9796.

Anorexia Nervosa and Related Eating Disorders Inc (ANRED). PO Box 5102, Eugene OR 97405. 541-344-1144.

Association for the Health Enrichment of Large People (AHELP). PO Drawer C, Radford VA 24743. 540-731-1778.

Chicago Center for Overcoming Overeating. PO Box 48, Deerfield IL 60015. 708-853-1200.

Council on Size & Weight Discrimination. PO Box 305, Mt. Marion NY 12456. 914-679-1209, 914-679-1206 (fax).

Diet/Weight Liberation. G-18 Anabel Taylor Hall, Cornell University, Ithaca NY 14853. 607-257-0563.

Largely Positive. PO Box 17223, Glendale WI 53217.

Largesse. 74 Woolsey St, PO Box 9404, New Haven CT 06534-0404. 203-787-1624 (fax and phone)

National Association to Advance Fat Acceptance (NAAFA). PO Box 188620, Sacramento CA 95818. 800-442-1214, 916-558-6881 (fax).

National Center for Overcoming Overeating. 315 W 86th St, 17B, New York NY 10024. 212-875-0442, 800-299-0577.

World Service Office of Overeaters Anonymous. PO Box 44020, Rio Rancho NM 87174-4020. 505-891-2664, 505-891-4320 (fax).

RECOMMENDED AUDIO AND VIDEO

Anorexia & Bulimia: The Silent Struggle, 1990. Produced and directed by Rebecca Ruggles Radcliffe. Eating Awareness Services and Education (EASE) PO Box 8032, Minneapolis MN 55408-0032. 612-825-7681, 612-891-4360 (fax). 29 minutes. Videocassette.

Body Image: Affirming Meditations for People of All Sizes, 1996. Whole Person Associates, 210 West Michigan, Duluth MN 55802-1908. 800-247-6789, 218-727-0505 (fax). 50 minutes. Audiocassette.

Body Trust: Undieting Your Way to Health and Happiness, 1993. Created by Dayle Hayes, RD. Produced by Production West Inc, 1001 S 24th St W, Billings MT 59102. 406-656-9417. 60 minutes. Videocassette.

Chair Dancing®: A New Concept in Aerobics Fitness, 1991. Created and choreographed by Jodi Stolove. Chair Dancing® International Inc, 2640 Del Mar Heights Rd, Suite 183, Del Mar CA 92014. 800-551-4FUN. 45 minutes and 10 minutes. Videocassette and audiocassette.

Eating: Guided Imagery for Making Peace with Food, 1996. Whole Person Associates, 210 West Michigan, Duluth MN 55802-1908. 800-247-6789, 218-727-0505 (fax). 50 minutes. Audiocassette.

The Enlightened Eating Tape Series, 1993. Produced and directed by Rebecca Ruggles Radcliffe. Eating Awareness Services and Education (EASE), PO Box 8032, Minneapolis MN 55408-0032. 612-825-7681. 60 minutes each. 6 audiocassettes.

The Famine Within, 1990. Developed by Katherine Gilday. Distributed by Direct Cinema Ltd, PO Box 10003, Santa Monica CA 90410-1003. 800-242-0000, 310-396-3223. 118 minutes. Videocassette.

Fat Chance, 1994. Produced by the Canadian National Film Board. VHS available from National Association to Advance Fat Acceptance (NAAFA) Book Service. 916-558-6880, 916-558-6881 (fax). 70 minutes. Videocassette.

Killing Us Softly: Advertising's Image of Women, 1979. Written by Jean Kilbourne. Cambridge Documentary Films Inc, PO Box 385, Cambridge MA 02139. 617-354-3677, 617-492-7653 (fax). 28 minutes. Videocassette.

The Losing Game, 1993. Produced and directed by Judy Cohen. Allbritton TV Productions, 3007 Tilden Street NW, Washington DC 20008. 202-364-7781, 202-364-7889 (fax). 50 minutes. Videocassette.

Making Healthy Choices: A Comprehensive 6-Session Video Course, 1995. Whole Person Associates, 210 W Michigan, Duluth MN 55802-1908. 1-800-247-6789, 218-727-0505 (fax). 20 minutes each. 6 videocassettes.

Overcoming Overeating: A Revolutionary Approach to Curing Eating Problems: A Full-Day Introductory Workshop, 1992. Jane R. Hirschmann and Carol H. Munter. National Center for Overcoming Overeating, Old Chelsea Station, Box 2757, New York NY 10113-0920. 800-299-0577. 5.5 hours. 4 audiocassettes.

Skin Deep: A Story about Eating Disorders, 1993. Disney Educational Productions, 105 Terry Drive, Suite 120, Newton PA 18940. 800-295-5010. 26 minutes. Videocassette.

Still Killing Us Softly: Advertising's Image of Women, 1987. Written by Jean Kilbourne. Cambridge Documentary Films Inc, PO Box 385, Cambridge MA 02139. 617-354-3677, 617-492-7653 (fax). 32 minutes. Videocassette.

Yoga for Round Bodies, Volumes 1 and *2,* 1995. Produced and directed by Linda DeMarco and Genia Pauli Haddon, Certified Kripalu Yoga Teachers. Plus Publications, Box 265, Suite 499, Scotland CT 06264. 800-793-0666. 90 minutes each. 2 videocassettes.

CONTRIBUTORS

Martha Belknap, MA. 1170 Dixon Road, Gold Hill, Boulder CO 80302. 303-447-9642. Marti is an educational consultant who specializes in creative relaxation and stress management skills. She has 30 years of teaching experience at all levels. Marti offers relaxation workshops and creativity courses through schools, universities, hospitals, and businesses. She is the author of *Taming Your Dragons,* and *Taming More Dragons,* two books and an audiocassette of creative relaxation activities for home and school.

Roxanne Bijold, MSE, RD. St. Mary's Medical Center, 407 E Third St, Duluth MN 55805. 218-726-4593. Roxanne is a registered dietitian with ten years of experience counseling clients with eating disorders, weight issues, diabetes, and heart disease. She has given numerous group presentations on healthy eating, behavior change, and body image. She has taught heart-healthy cooking classes and is involved in the nutrition education of medical students and residents.

Richard Boyum, EdD. Senior Psychologist, University of Wisconsin–Eau Claire, Eau Claire WI 54702. 715-836-5521 (w), 715-874-6222 (h). Dr. Boyum has been a practicing psychologist, counselor, and teacher at UW–Eau Claire since 1973. His specialities include the use of guided imagery and metaphor in creating healthier behaviors. He also works with individuals, families, and organizations in creating behavioral changes through the use of both individual and systems models.

Lucia Capacchione, MA, PhD. PO Box 1355, Cambria CA 93428. 310-281-7495 (w), 805-546-1424 (h). Lucia is an art therapist, seminar leader, and corporate consultant. She is the author of nine books, including *The Creative Journal* (with versions for adults, teens, and children); *The Well-Being Journal; Lighten Up Your Body, Lighten Up Your Life* (coauthored with Elizabeth Johnson and James Strohecker); and *The Picture of Health*. After healing herself from a collagen disease through creative journaling, Lucia has dedicated her professional life to researching right brain approaches to healing and empowering individuals and organizations with new vision and innovative healing alternatives. Her best-known books, *The Power of Your Other Hand* and *Recovery of your Inner Child,* open new doors to self-health.

Sandy Stewart Christian, MSW. Editor, Product Development Team, Whole Person Associates, 210 West Michigan, Duluth MN 55802. 218-727-0500 (w), 218-728-3916 (h). Editor of *Volume 5* of *Structured Exercises in Stress Management* and *Wellness Promotion,* Sandy is a licensed independent clinical social worker and a licensed marriage and family therapist. In her work as a therapist, teacher, trainer, and consultant, Sandy has maintained a lively whole person focus in health and stress management.

Cheri K. Erdman, EdD. College of DuPage, 22nd and Lambert Rd, Glen Elleyn IL 60137. 708-942-2059. Cheri is author of the book, *Nothing to Lose: A Guide to Sane Living in a Larger Body* (HarperCollins, 1995). Her doctoral dissertation was on the process of body-size acceptance in large women. Cheri taught her first Women and Body Image course in 1981. She continues this work as well as teaching courses, facilitating workshops, and sponsoring retreats promoting fitness and self-esteem for large women. She considers herself to be a healthy, fit, sane, smart, sexy, creative, happy, fat woman and is on a mission to influence other larger women to feel the same.

Laura K. Field, MA. Chevron Corporation, 2005 Diamond Blvd, Room 2130N/Section 270, Concord CA 94520. 510-680-3313. Laura is the Health Promotion Specialist for the Chevron Corporation in Concord CA where she designs health education programming for Chevron employees in the San Francisco Bay area. Her classes and workshops in exercise adherence, eating behavior, body image, goal setting, conflict resolution, communication skills, stress reduction, and coping with organizational transition have earned her a reputation as a dynamic and insightful speaker. Her written work has been published in a number of professional journals including *The American Journal for Health Promotion.* Laura provides consultation services to both individuals and corporations who are seeking both personal and organizational wellness.

Mary Graff, MSW, LICSW. Lake Superior Associates, 700 Sellwood Building, 202 W Superior St, Duluth MN 55802. 218-726-1006. Mary is a clinical social worker in a small, private group practice with a speciality in trauma recovery issues and marriage and family therapy. She has worked in the area of mental health for over 23 years and has taught courses at University of Minnesota–Duluth and University of Wisconsin–Superior Social Work departments on Family Systems Theory, Women and Social Policy, Social Work in a Clinical Setting, and Process in Clinical Social Work.

Chris Henley, MS. Licensed Psychologist, Lake Superior Associates, 700 Sellwood Building, 202 W Superior St, Duluth MN 55802. 218-726-1006. Chris is a psychologist working clinically with adults and adolescents with eating disorders. Working in this field for many years, she has designed, implemented, and directed three separate eating disorders programs for adolescents and young adults. Her passion is helping young women find their voices and thus prevent eating disorders. She also speaks and conducts clinical training in eating disorders and other clinical issues.

Nancy Hinzman, COTA. Mental Health Services, St. Luke's Hospital of Duluth, 915 E First St, Duluth MN 55805. 218-726-5237. Nancy is a certified Occupational Therapy Assistant working in St. Luke's Inpatient, Outpatient, Partial Hospitalization, and Eating Disorders Treatment programs. She also works with a men's group. Her specialities are working with body image, feelings, and self-awareness using artistic mediums such as drawing and painting.

Jane R. Hirschmann, MSW. National Center for Overcoming Overeating, 315 W 86th St, Suite 17B, New York NY 10024. 212-875-0442. Jane is a psychotherapist in private practice specializing in treating women and children with eating problems. With Carol H. Munter, she is coauthor of *When Women Stop Hating Their Bodies* (Fawcett, 1995) and *Overcoming Overeating* (Fawcett, 1988). With Lela Zaphiropoulos, she is coauthor of *Preventing Childhood Eating Problems* (Gurze, 1994). Jane is also the President of the National Center for Overcoming Overeating, an organization committed to putting an end to body hatred and dieting.

Marcia Germaine Hutchinson, EdD. 88 W Goulding St, Sherborn MA 01770. 508-653-3665. Dr. Marcia Germaine Hutchinson is a Licensed Psychologist in private practice in the Boston area and is the author of the pioneering book, *Transforming Body Image: Learning to Love the Body You Have* (Crossing Press, 1985). She is noted for her creative and powerful use of therapeutic imagery. Dr. Hutchinson is an internationally recognized pioneer in the treatment of body image and has presented her *Transforming Body Image* workshop throughout the US and Canada.

Joanne P. Ikeda, MA, RD. Department of Nutritional Sciences, Cooperative Extension Office, Morgan Hall, Room 9A #3104, Berkeley CA 94720. 510-642-2790. Joanne is the Cooperative Extension Nutrition Education Specialist and a lecturer in the Department of Nutritional Sciences at the University of California–Berkeley. She conducts in-service training for health professionals on preventing and treating pediatric obesity. She is the author of the book, *Am I Fat: Helping Young Children Accept Difference in Body Size.*

Carol Johnson, MA. Largely Positive, PO Box 17223, Glendale, WI 53217. 414-224-0404. Carol is a *magna cum laude* graduate of Kent State University with bachelor's and master's degrees in sociology. She is also a certified therapist and author of the book, *Self-Esteem Comes in All Sizes: How to Be Happy and Healthy at Your Natural Weight* (Doubleday, 1995). Her organization, Largely Positive Inc, is dedicated to promoting health, self-esteem, and well-being among larger people. She presents workshops on self-esteem and size acceptance to both professional and consumer groups and is currently helping to organize Largely Positive support groups throughout the country. (Persons interested in starting a group may write to her at the address above.)

Susan Kano. 18 Holiday Rd, Wayland ME 01778. 508-358-4811. Susan is an author, lecturer, and workshop leader who specializes in the field of weight control and eating disorders. Her groundbreaking book, *Making Peace with Food,* offers a holistic self-help program for anorexics, bulimics, and yo-yo dieters of all sizes. Susan has been leading workshops for chronic dieters and eating disorder sufferers since 1980 and has received the Walkley Prize for empirical research on body image, eating patterns, and associated conflicts, from Wesleyan University. She has repeatedly appeared on television and radio to discuss eating disorders and natural weight control. Susan is currently collaborating on a book with photographer Patrica Schwarz using art and portrait photography to promote positive body image among women.

Julie Waltz Kembel, MSEd, CHES. 5728 North Via Umbrosa, Tucson AZ 85750. 520/ 229-8435. Julie is a counselor, health educator, author, workshop leader, and national speaker who specializes in innovative, behavioral approaches to wellness. Julie is the author of the award-winning book, *Winning the Weight and Wellness Game* (Northwest Learning Associates, 1993). Other titles include, *No Ifs, Ands, or Butts: A Smoker's Guide to Kicking the Habit* and *ROLE Play: Personalities in Action.* Julie and her work have been featured in national publications and televised special reports. Julie serves on the Advisory Board of *Vitality* magazine and is currently the Education Director of the Health and Healing Center at the world-famous Canyon Ranch Resort in Tucson AZ.

Laura Loving, MDiv. 515 Brasted Place, Waukesha WI 53186. 414-547-4140. Laura is a minister in the United Church of Christ. She graduated from Smith College with a BA in Art History and from Princeton Theological Seminary with a Masters of Divinity. She has served churches throughout the Upper Midwest and has specialized in interim ministry and a ministry of workshop and retreat leadership. With emphasis on the playful and the prayerful, Laura's retreats and workshops feed the spirit while offering thanks to the Holy Spirit for the great gifts of humor, creativity, spontaneity, and grace.

© 1996 WHOLE PERSON PRESS 210 WEST MICHIGAN DULUTH MN 55802 ∎(800) 247-6789

Pat Lyons, RN, MA. 416 Lester Ave, Oakland CA 94606. 510-763-7365. Pat is a lifelong sports enthusiast and coauthor of *Great Shape: The First Fitness Guide for Large Women.* She has also written chapters in three other books related to fitness, body image, weight discrimination, health care access, and women's health. She is a leader in the non-dieting/size acceptance movement, a frequent speaker at conferences, and her work has been featured in numerous radio, TV, and print media stories. Currently she is a Regional Health Education Consultant at Kaiser Permanente, Northern California Region.

Mary L. Martin, PhD, LP. Lake Superior Associates, 700 Sellwood Building, Duluth MN 55802. 218-726-1006. Mary is a clinical psychologist in a small group practice. She specializes in posttraumatic work, eating disorders, mood disorders, and personal growth development. In her 32 years of experience, Mary has worked in mental health settings, directed an outreach program for children and families, and consulted with hospital mental health services and private counseling agencies.

Carol H. Munter. National Center for Overcoming Overeating, 315 W 86th St, Suite 17B, New York NY 10024. 212-875-0442. Carol is a psychoanalyst in private practice in New York City. Her interest in developing a methodology for the treatment of compulsive eating began when, to deal with her own struggle, she started the first antidieting group for women in 1970. With Jane R. Hirschmann, she is the coauthor of *When Women Stop Hating Their Bodies* (Fawcett, 1995) and *Overcoming Overeating* (Fawcett, 1988). She is the codirector of the National Center for Overcoming Overeating and a Certified Eating Disorders Specialist.

Gayle Potter, RN, C. Partial Hospitalization Program, St. Luke's Hospital of Duluth, 915 E First St, Duluth MN 55805. 218-726-5237 (w). Gayle is currently employed at St. Luke's Hospital of Duluth in the Adult Partial Hospitalization Program working with women with depression, posttraumatic stress disorder, anxiety disorders, relationship and self-esteem issues. Her background is in both inpatient and outpatient mental health settings.

Yvonne Prettner, MA. Program Coordinator, St. Luke's Hospital Eating Disorders Center, 915 E First St, Duluth MN 55805. 218-726-5506. Yvonne is a licensed psychologist who began working with addictions in 1978 and has worked with eating disorders since 1981. She has designed and run outpatient, partial hospitalization, and residential recovery programs for women. In addition, she has a clinical practice with competencies in posttraumatic stress, dissociative disorders, adult survivor, sexuality, and gender role issues.

Sandy Queen. Director, LIFEWORKS Inc, PO Box 2668, Columbia MD 21045. 410-796-5310. Sandy is the founder and director of LIFEWORKS Inc, a training/counseling firm that specializes in helping people take a better look at their lives through humor, laughter, and play. She has developed many innovative programs in the areas of stress-reduction, humor, children's wellness, and self-esteem.

Rebecca Ruggles Radcliffe. Eating Awareness Services and Education (EASE), PO Box 8032, Minneapolis MN 55408-0032. 800-470-4769 or 612-825-7681. Rebecca lectures nationally and conducts workshops on women's issues, body image, emotional eating, self-esteem, personal growth, and related issues. Rebecca is especially gifted at putting emotional issues that cause overeating into everyday language and creating exercises for personal change. She is the author of *Enlightened Eating: Understanding and Changing Your Relationship with Food* and *The Enlightened Newsletter,* as well as other materials for positive lifestyle change.

Geneen Roth. PO Box 2852, Santa Cruz CA 95063. 408-685-8601. Geneen is a writer and teacher who gained international prominence through her work in the field of eating disorders. She is the founder of Breaking Free Workshops, which she has been leading since 1979. She is author of four books entitled *Feeding the Hungry Heart, Breaking Free from Compulsive Eating, Whey Weight?* and *The New York Times* best-seller *When Food is Love.* Geneen's newest book *APPETITES: On the Search for True Nourishment* will be released in April 1996. Geneen has appeared on *The Oprah Winfrey Show, 20/20,* and the *NBC Nightly News.* Her work has been featured in *New Age Journal, The New York Times, Cosmopolitan,* and *The Chicago Tribune.*

Mary O'Brien Sippel, RN, MS. Licensed Psychologist, 22 E St. Andrews, Duluth MN 55803. 218-723-6130 (w), 218-724-5935 (h). Mary has spent over twenty-five years working in the field of community health and education. Her experience in teaching stress management, burnout prevention, and wellness promotion across the country has enabled her to be her own best caretaker as career woman, wife, and mother of two teenagers. Mary is currently a personal counselor and adjunct faculty member at the College of St. Scholastica in Duluth MN. She has ten publications to her credit. Mary never tires of sharing her enthusiasm for life, both on paper and in front of her audiences.

Pam Solberg-Tapper, MT. Director, Miller-Dwan New Direction Center, 502 E Second St, Duluth MN 55805. 218-720-1165. As Director of Miller-Dwan New Direction Center's Weight Management and Health Promotion/Disease Prevention Program, Pam leads a multidisciplinary team of physicians, nurses, dietitians, master's level behavioral counselors, and exercise physiologists. Pam develops and implements wellness programming for hospitals, businesses, and schools. She promotes healthy lifestyles as a contributing writer for a local newspaper and as a member of Toastmasters and Rotary International in her community.

Katherine H. Speare, PhD. Center for Psychological Health, 1507 Tower Ave, Suite 210B, Superior WI 54880. 715-394-2920. Katherine is a licensed psychologist with over 20 years experience. In her private practice, Dr. Speare specializes in working with adult women on depression and related issues. For over five years, she has been presenting workshops on boundaries to medical professionals, psychologists, psychotherapists, social service workers, clergy, law enforcement, and chemical dependency professionals. She has provided consultation to various staff groups who are experiencing boundary-related problems. She has recently developed and has been presenting a workshop on Women at Mid-life and is currently pursuing research on creativity.

Jodi Stolove, MS. Chair Dancing® International Inc, 2640 Del Mar Heights Rd, Suite 183, Del Mar CA 92014. 800-551-4FUN. Jodi has been dancing since she was a child and has taught ballet, tap, jazz, and ballroom dance for the past 14 years. A *cum laude* graduate of the University of Michigan, with a BA in Dance and Education, her teaching skills have been enriched by her Masters in Counseling Psychology. She invented the Chair Dancing® concept when she fractured her ankle and taught dance sitting in a chair. Creativity born of necessity resulted in her development of a unique fitness program combining the pleasure of exercise, dance, and music. Chair Dancing® has been featured nationally on *Today* (NBC) and *CBS This Morning*.

Ruth Strom McCutcheon, RN-CANP, MSN. Director of Nursing Operations, Duluth Clinic, 400 E Third St, Duluth MN 55805. 218-722-8364. Ruth is a nurse practitioner specializing in women's health care whose work for over fifteen years counseling groups and individuals in the area of eating disorders led her back to graduate school in psych/mental health nursing. Ruth has recently traded the creative opportunities of providing health care services to college students for the challenge of assisting a thriving regional clinic to make a healthy transition to managed care.

Sally Strosahl, MA. Marriage and Family Therapist, 116 S Westlawn, Aurora IL 60506. 708-897-9796. Sally received an MA in clinical psychology, trained at the Wholistic Health Center, and researched the relationship between stress and illness. In addition to her private practice in marriage and family therapy, Sally frequently presents workshops in the areas of stress and wellness management, burnout prevention, body image and size acceptance, and marriage enrichment. She particularly enjoys working with *systems* (family, work groups, agencies, businesses, churches) to help enhance each member's growth and well-being. She is the cofounder of ABUNDIA, a service providing size-acceptance training to professionals and other groups.

Larry Tobin, MA. Jade Mist Press, 1002 Maple Way, Stevenson WA 98648. 509-427-7082. Larry is a special educator, school psychologist, and national trainer on working with troubled children. He has authored *What Do You Do with a Child Like This?; 62 Ways to Create Change in the Lives of Troubled Children*; and *Time Well Spent,* a yearlong stress management planner.

John W Travis, MD, MPH. 21489 Orr Springs Rd, Ukiah CA 95482. 707-937-2331. John is the founder of the first Wellness Center, author of *The Wellness Inventory* and coauthor of *Wellness: Small Changes You Can Use to Make a Big Difference, Wellness for Helping Professionals*, and *A Change of Heart: A Global Wellness Inventory*. His commitment is to provide safe spaces, conflict resolution skills, and the experiences of cooperation and partnership for helping professionals—replacing the authoritarian mindset of the illness-care industry and the culture at large.

Nancy Loving Tubesing, MEd, EdD. Product Development Director, Whole Person Associates, 210 West Michigan, Duluth MN 55802. 218-727-0500 (w), 218-724-7014 (h). With her roots and training in education, group counseling, creative problem solving, medicine, and theology, Nancy brings a truly whole person perspective to her teaching and writing. The soothing voice on most Whole Person relaxation tapes belongs to this author of *Seeking Your Healthy Balance* and senior editor of the *Structured Exercises in Stress Management* and *Wellness Promotion* series.

TOOLS FOR FOOD AND BODY CONNECTIONS

WORKING WITH GROUPS TO EXPLORE FOOD & BODY CONNECTIONS
Sandy Stewart Christian, MSW, Editor

36 group processes gathered from experts around the country tackle complex and painful issues nearly everyone is concerned about—dieting, weight, healthy eating, fitness, body image, and self-esteem.

❑ **Working with Groups to Explore Food & Body Connections / $24.95**
❑ **Worksheet Masters / $9.95**

EATING: Visualizations for Making Peace with Food

Relax . . . and imagine your way to healthy, joy-filled eating! Five meditations to help you make peace with food, tune in to your body and its hungers, soothe eating anxieties, and trust yourself to make healthy choices. Music by Steven Halpern.

Side A: Mealtime Meditation, Empty/Full (25:00)
Side B: Food & Moods, Wholesome Feasts, Sensory Awareness (25:00)

❑ **Eating audiotape / $11.95**

BODY IMAGE: Affirming Meditations for People of All Sizes

Learn to love and accept the body you have. Listen, respect, and trust its messages. Six relaxing and affirming visualizations promote positive self-image, size-acceptance, and personal empowerment—no matter what your size or shape. Music by Steven Eckels.

Side A: Relaxing Breath, Virtual Body, Body Talk (25:00)
Side B: Cleansing Breath, Magic Pill, Mind Mirror Breathing (25:00)

❑ **Body Image audiotape / $11.95**

WORKSHEET MASTERS
Complete packages of (8 1/2" x 11") photocopy masters are available for most Whole Person working with groups volumes, including

Exploring Food & Body Connections
Working with Women's Groups
Structured Exercises in Wellness Promotion
Working with Groups to Overcome Panic, Anxiety, & Phobias

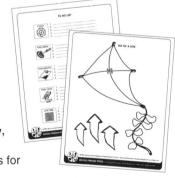

Use the masters for easy duplication of handouts for each participant. $9.95 per volume.

❑ **Exploring Food & Body Connection Worksheets / $9.95**
❑ **Working with Women's Groups Worksheets / $9.95 per volume**
❑ **Structured Exercises in Wellness Promotion Worksheets / $9.95 per volume**
❑ **Working with Groups to Overcome Panic, Anxiety, & Phobias Worksheets / $9.95**

© 1996 WHOLE PERSON PRESS 210 WEST MICHIGAN DULUTH MN 55802 ■ (800) 247-6789